Challenges and Perspectives of Neurological Disorders

Challenges and Perspectives of Neurological Disorders

Editors

Woon-Man Kung
Dina Nur Anggraini Ningrum

MDPI • Basel • Beijing • Wuhan • Barcelona • Belgrade • Manchester • Tokyo • Cluj • Tianjin

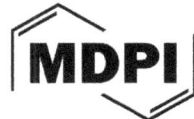

Editors
Woon-Man Kung
Division of Neurosurgery,
Department of Surgery,
Taipei Tzu Chi Hospital,
Buddhist Tzu Chi Medical
Foundation,
New Taipei City,
Taiwan

Dina Nur Anggraini
Ningrum
Public Health Department,
Faculty of Sport Sciences,
Universitas Negeri Semarang,
Semarang City,
Indonesia

Editorial Office
MDPI
St. Alban-Anlage 66
4052 Basel, Switzerland

This is a reprint of articles from the Special Issue published online in the open access journal *Brain Sciences* (ISSN 2076-3425) (available at: www.mdpi.com/journal/brainsci/special_issues/Challenges_Perspectives_Neurological_Disorders).

For citation purposes, cite each article independently as indicated on the article page online and as indicated below:

LastName, A.A.; LastName, B.B.; LastName, C.C. Article Title. *Journal Name* **Year**, *Volume Number*, Page Range.

ISBN 978-3-0365-7503-2 (Hbk)
ISBN 978-3-0365-7502-5 (PDF)

© 2023 by the authors. Articles in this book are Open Access and distributed under the Creative Commons Attribution (CC BY) license, which allows users to download, copy and build upon published articles, as long as the author and publisher are properly credited, which ensures maximum dissemination and a wider impact of our publications.
The book as a whole is distributed by MDPI under the terms and conditions of the Creative Commons license CC BY-NC-ND.

Contents

About the Editors vii

Preface to "Challenges and Perspectives of Neurological Disorders" ix

Dina Nur Anggraini Ningrum and Woon-Man Kung
Challenges and Perspectives of Neurological Disorders
Reprinted from: *Brain Sci.* 2023, *13*, 676, doi:10.3390/brainsci13040676 1

Mengxia Wan, Ji He, Junyan Huo, Can Sun, Yu Fu and Dongsheng Fan
Intermediate-Length GGC Repeat Expansion in NOTCH2NLC Was Identified in Chinese Patients with Amyotrophic Lateral Sclerosis
Reprinted from: *Brain Sci.* 2023, *13*, 85, doi:10.3390/brainsci13010085 5

Qian Zhou, Meiqun Tian, Huan Yang and Yue-Bei Luo
Adult-Onset Neuronal Intranuclear Inclusion Disease with Mitochondrial Encephalomyopathy, Lactic Acidosis, and Stroke-Like (MELAS-like) Episode: A Case Report and Review of Literature
Reprinted from: *Brain Sci.* 2022, *12*, 1377, doi:10.3390/brainsci12101377 15

Antigoni Avramouli, Marios G. Krokidis, Themis P. Exarchos and Panagiotis Vlamos
In Silico Structural Analysis Predicting the Pathogenicity of PLP1 Mutations in Multiple Sclerosis
Reprinted from: *Brain Sci.* 2022, *13*, 42, doi:10.3390/brainsci13010042 27

Fangyang Jiao, Min Wang, Xiaoming Sun, Zizhao Ju, Jiaying Lu and Luyao Wang et al.
Based on Tau PET Radiomics Analysis for the Classification of Alzheimer's Disease and Mild Cognitive Impairment
Reprinted from: *Brain Sci.* 2023, *13*, 367, doi:10.3390/brainsci13020367 41

Juanjuan Jiang, Jieming Zhang, Chenyang Li, Zhihua Yu, Zhuangzhi Yan and Jiehui Jiang
Development of a Machine Learning Model to Discriminate Mild Cognitive Impairment Subjects from Normal Controls in Community Screening
Reprinted from: *Brain Sci.* 2022, *12*, 1149, doi:10.3390/brainsci12091149 55

Yan Zhao, Jieming Zhang, Yue Chen and Jiehui Jiang
A Novel Deep Learning Radiomics Model to Discriminate AD, MCI and NC: An Exploratory Study Based on Tau PET Scans from ADNI [†]
Reprinted from: *Brain Sci.* 2022, *12*, 1067, doi:10.3390/brainsci12081067 67

Zizhao Ju, Zhuoyuan Li, Jiaying Lu, Fangyang Jiao, Huamei Lin and Weiqi Bao et al.
In Vivo Tau Burden Is Associated with Abnormal Brain Functional Connectivity in Alzheimer's Disease: A ^{18}F-Florzolotau Study
Reprinted from: *Brain Sci.* 2022, *12*, 1355, doi:10.3390/brainsci12101355 81

Cheng-Chi Lee, Jeng-Fu You, Yu-Chi Wang, Shao-Wei Lan, Kuo-Chen Wei and Ko-Ting Chen et al.
Gross Total Resection Promotes Subsequent Recovery and Further Enhancement of Impaired Natural Killer Cell Activity in Glioblastoma Patients
Reprinted from: *Brain Sci.* 2022, *12*, 1144, doi:10.3390/brainsci12091144 93

Tingyu Yi, Alai Zhan, Yanmin Wu, Yimin Li, Xiufen Zheng and Dinglai Lin et al.
Endovascular Treatment of ICAS Patients: Targeting Reperfusion Rather than Residual Stenosis
Reprinted from: *Brain Sci.* 2022, *12*, 966, doi:10.3390/brainsci12080966 107

Vittorio Riso, Tommaso Filippo Nicoletti, Salvatore Rossi, Maria Gabriella Vita, Perna Alessia and Daniele Di Natale et al.
Neurological Erdheim–Chester Disease Manifesting with Subacute or Progressive Cerebellar Ataxia: Novel Case Series and Review of the Literature
Reprinted from: *Brain Sci.* **2022**, *13*, 26, doi:10.3390/brainsci13010026 . . . . **117**

Hyuk-June Moon and Sungmin Han
Perspective: Present and Future of Virtual Reality for Neurological Disorders
Reprinted from: *Brain Sci.* **2022**, *12*, 1692, doi:10.3390/brainsci12121692 . . . . **129**

About the Editors

Woon-Man Kung

Woon-Man Kung received his M.D. degree from the School of Medicine, Taipei Medical University (TMU), Taipei, Taiwan, in 1999. In 2012, he received his M.Sc. degree in Biomedical Engineering from the College of Medicine and College of Engineering, National Taiwan University (NTU), Taipei, Taiwan. Dr. Kung now serves as a Consultant Neurosurgeon in the Division of Neurosurgery, Department of Surgery, Taipei Tzu Chi Hospital (TCH), Buddhist Tzu Chi Medical Foundation, New Taipei City, Taiwan, as well as an Adjunct Associate Professor in the Department of Exercise and Health Promotion, College of Kinesiology and Health, Chinese Culture University (CCU), Taipei, Taiwan. He also holds International Membership of the professional association at the Congress of Neurological Surgeons (CNS), USA. He currently works on the Editorial/Advisory Board of several indexed journals and acts as an ad hoc reviewer for a number of prestigious scientific journals.

Dina Nur Anggraini Ningrum

Dina obtained her B.S.P.H. (Epidemiology) degree in 2004 from Diponegoro University, Indonesia. In 2013, she received her M.P.H. degree from Diponegoro University, Indonesia, in the field of Health Informatics. Then, in 2022, she obtained her Ph.D. from the Graduate Institute of Biomedical Informatics, College of Medical Science and Technology, Taipei Medical University, Taiwan. She is currently an Assistant Professor in the Public Health Department at Semarang State University, Indonesia. She is a collaborator for Global Burden Diseases and is interested in issues related to disease/health problem prediction using big data and artificial intelligence technology, digital epidemiology, and health informatics. She is also a reviewer of several reputable international journals and is the editor of journals indexed by Scopus.

Preface to "Challenges and Perspectives of Neurological Disorders"

This Special Issue reprint consists of 11 articles published in *Brain Sciences* from a call for papers on the topic of "Challenges and Perspectives of Neurological Disorders", which welcomed contributions from various disciplines and perspectives on this important and timely field.

Neurological disorders are one of the most significant issues in medicine and public health today. They affect a large population worldwide and place a huge burden on society and the economy. However, there are still many challenges and gaps in the prevention, diagnosis, treatment, and rehabilitation of neurological disorders. Therefore, there is a need for more information and knowledge sharing among different disciplines and stakeholders.

The purpose of this Special Issue is to offer a comprehensive and in-depth understanding of the current situation and future development of neurological disorders. It explores various aspects of neurological disorders, from basic science to clinical practice, and examines the mechanisms, genetics, markers, images, surgeries, lifestyle changes, and other topics of neurological disorders.

The target audience for this Special Issue is anyone who is interested in or involved in the field of neurological disorders. The authors involved in this Special Issue are distinguished experts who have shared their valuable insights and experiences on various topics of neurological disorders.

We would like to express our sincere gratitude to all the authors, reviewers, and the editorial team of the journal for their excellent work and cooperation.

Woon-Man Kung and Dina Nur Anggraini Ningrum
Editors

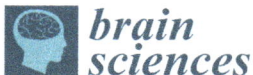

Editorial

Challenges and Perspectives of Neurological Disorders

Dina Nur Anggraini Ningrum [1] and Woon-Man Kung [2,3,*]

1. Public Health Department, Faculty of Sport Sciences, Universitas Negeri Semarang, Semarang 50229, Indonesia
2. Division of Neurosurgery, Department of Surgery, Taipei Tzu Chi Hospital, Buddhist Tzu Chi Medical Foundation, New Taipei City 23142, Taiwan
3. Department of Exercise and Health Promotion, College of Kinesiology and Health, Chinese Culture University, Taipei 11114, Taiwan
* Correspondence: nskungwm@yahoo.com.tw

Neurological disorders pose significant challenges to healthcare systems worldwide. These conditions can severely impact an individual's quality of life, leading to physical, emotional, and cognitive impairments [1]. Managing neurological disorders often requires specialized care, including access to medical experts, various diagnostic tools, and complicated treatment options. Unfortunately, most real-world scenarios lack sufficient resources to provide adequate care to patients with neurological disorders. Furthermore, the complexity of these conditions makes diagnosis and treatment difficult, leading to misdiagnosis and delayed care, which can exacerbate symptoms and increase the burden on patients and caregivers [2]. Addressing these challenges requires a comprehensive approach that includes improving access to care, investing in research to advance diagnostic and treatment options, and increasing public awareness of neurological disorders [3]. The articles contained in this Special Issue highlight significant advances and encourage further investigational efforts in this exciting field.

The hereditary etiology of neuronal intranuclear inclusion disease (NIID) and its existence in other neurodegenerative disorders is an interesting theme. A study by Wan et al. screened 476 individuals with amyotrophic lateral sclerosis (ALS) and 210 individuals without ALS for the manifestation of a GGC repeat expansion in the Notch Homolog 2 N-terminal-like C gene (NOTCH2NLC). The outcomes indicated that intermediate NOTCH2NLC GGC repeat expansion was connected with Chinese patients with ALS [4].

Zhou et al. reported a rare case report of an individual with NIID who presented with mitochondrial encephalomyopathy, lactic acidosis, and stroke-like (MELAS-like) symptoms, as well as reversible brain magnetic resonance imaging (MRI) diffusion-weighted imaging (DWI) hyperintensities. The diagnosis of this presented case was determined through skin biopsy in addition to genetic testing, in which a steroid treatment resulted in improved symptoms and neuroimaging. This article emphasizes the importance of distinguishing NIID from MELAS and the potential for reversible DWI hyperintensities in NIID [5].

Avramouli's laboratory analyzed the role of proteolipid protein (PLP) 1 missense point mutations in the pathogenicity of multiple sclerosis (MS). Computational structural biology methods were applied for the evaluation of these mutation effects on the structural stability and flexibility of PLP1. This study demonstrated that the vast majority of variants can change the functionality of protein structures, and in silico genomic methods were likewise carried out to predict the importance of these mutations related to protein functionality. The study suggests that a better description of therapeutic applications and clinical strategies in patients with MS can be achieved by further research into the impact of these mutations [6].

Jiao et al. used radiomics analysis to improve classification accuracy in individuals with Alzheimer's disease (AD) and mild cognitive impairment (MCI). They aimed to identify high-order features from pathological biomarkers and to improve classification accuracy based on tau positron emission tomography (PET) images. Distinct cohorts were

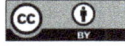

used in the study, and the radiomics features of tau PET imaging of AD-related brain regions were computed for classification using a support vector machine (SVM) model. The model was trained and validated in the first cohort and tested in the second. The results showed that Tau PET radiomics analysis offers a perspective to anticipate clinical diagnosis as well as to figure out risk factors in MCI patients [7].

The study proposed by Jiang et al. features a new machine learning (ML) analytical method that utilizes electroencephalography (EEG), eye tracking (ET), and neuropsychological assessments to screen for MCI in the community. The proposed model achieved high classification accuracy in both training and validation groups and in an independent test group. The proposed model also provided exceptional classification performances, advocating its capacity for subsequent use in predicting cognitive decline [8].

Besides the previously mentioned ML approach, this study proposed another novel model utilizing deep learning radiomics (DLR) by Zhao et al. to differentiate AD, MCI, and normal control (NC) subjects by tau PET scans. The DLR model performed the most outstanding classification performance, when compared to traditional models, thus demonstrating potential clinical value in discriminating AD, MCI, and NC [9].

Notably, the application of a new second-generation tau radiotracer, ^{18}F-Florzolotau, was investigated to estimate the association of regional tau accumulation and brain functional connectivity (FC) abnormalities in patients with AD and MCI. Additionally, the proportion loss of functional connectivity strength (PLFCS) was found to be a new indicator of brain FC alteration. In the research performed by Ju et al., the authors found that PLFCS and functional connection strength (FCs) were higher in the AD and MCI groups when compared to the normal control group. The study concludes that brain FC abnormality is correlated with tau pathology in AD and MCI [10].

In a clinical study, Lee et al. implied that natural killer activity (NKA) was significantly impaired in glioblastoma patients, but it recovered and was significantly enhanced on postoperative day (POD) 30, particularly in patients who underwent gross total resection (GTR) when compared to those who underwent subtotal resection (STR). The impaired NKA recovery was also associated with an increase in the $CD56^{bright}CD16^-$ NK cell subset. Therefore, the study suggests that GTR may improve NKA and increase the $CD56^{bright}CD16^-$ NK subset, which could be associated with subsequent patient prognosis, and should be performed when possible [11].

In the following research by Yi et al., the association of residual stenosis severity or reperfusion status with artery reocclusion following endovascular treatment for patients with middle cerebral artery (MCA) atherosclerotic ischemic occlusions was inspected. The authors showed that reperfusion status was significantly associated with intraprocedural reocclusion, and individuals experiencing effective thrombectomy reperfusion had a smaller proportion of intraprocedural occlusion regardless of residual stenosis severity. Moreover, once effective reperfusion was attained, the delayed reocclusion rate was relatively decreased and did not significantly differ between individuals with severe residual stenosis and patients with mild to moderate residual stenosis [12].

Riso's team investigated Erdheim–Chester disease (ECD), an unusual clonal disorder of histiocytic myeloid precursors depicted by multisystem involvement, and its neurological presentations. They retrospectively collected and described a small number of patients with ECD, all revealing cerebellar presentations. The ECD clinical neurological manifestation always includes cerebellar features, demonstrating a subacute or progressive course. The study suggests that recognizing ECD can be extremely challenging with certain unique expressions that are beneficial for addressing it [13].

Finally, it is important to notice that the accessibility of virtual reality (VR) technology for people with neurological disorders has not been explored extensively. An innovative perspective communication by Moon et al. suggests that future research should focus on expanding the use of VR technology for diagnostic purposes and studying its potential benefits in neurological disorders [14].

In summary, these articles reflect recent advances and explore the use of innovative technologies and techniques in the field of neurology. We aim to explore an updated advancement of scientific knowledge to improve patient care. In hope that this collection will not only stimulate further research studies, we expect researchers and clinicians to facilitate the importance of making these tools accessible to individuals with neurological disorders.

Author Contributions: D.N.A.N. wrote the draft. W.-M.K. reviewed and revised the manuscript. Both authors copyedited the language. All authors have read and agreed to the published version of the manuscript.

Acknowledgments: We would like to extend our heartfelt gratitude to the colleagues who contribute their innovative research to this Special Issue. Similarly, endless valuable inputs from reviewers and editors to confirm the high standards of the articles are appreciated. Finally, we would like to acknowledge the publisher, without their assistance, we would be unable to publish this impactful topic.

Conflicts of Interest: The authors declare no conflict of interest.

References

1. Thakur, K.T.; Albanese, E.; Giannakopoulos, P.; Jette, N.; Linde, M.; Prince, M.J.; Steiner, T.J.; Dua, T. Neurological Disorders. In *Mental, Neurological, and Substance Use Disorders: Disease Control Priorities*, 3rd ed.; Patel, V., Chisholm, D., Dua, T., Laxminarayan, R., Medina-Mora, M.E., Eds.; The International Bank for Reconstruction and Development/The World Bank: Washington, DC, USA, 2016; Volume 4.
2. Ganapathy, V.; Graham, G.D.; DiBonaventura, M.D.; Gillard, P.J.; Goren, A.; Zorowitz, R.D. Caregiver burden, productivity loss, and indirect costs associated with caring for patients with poststroke spasticity. *Clin. Interv. Aging* **2015**, *10*, 1793–1802. [CrossRef] [PubMed]
3. Feigin, V.L.; Vos, T.; Nichols, E.; Owolabi, M.O.; Carroll, W.M.; Dichgans, M.; Deuschl, G.; Parmar, P.; Brainin, M.; Murray, C. The global burden of neurological disorders: Translating evidence into policy. *Lancet Neurol.* **2020**, *19*, 255–265. [CrossRef] [PubMed]
4. Wan, M.; He, J.; Huo, J.; Sun, C.; Fu, Y.; Fan, D. Intermediate-Length GGC Repeat Expansion in NOTCH2NLC Was Identified in Chinese Patients with Amyotrophic Lateral Sclerosis. *Brain Sci.* **2023**, *13*, 85. [CrossRef] [PubMed]
5. Zhou, Q.; Tian, M.; Yang, H.; Luo, Y.B. Adult-Onset Neuronal Intranuclear Inclusion Disease with Mitochondrial Encephalomyopathy, Lactic Acidosis, and Stroke-Like (MELAS-like) Episode: A Case Report and Review of Literature. *Brain Sci.* **2022**, *12*, 1377. [CrossRef] [PubMed]
6. Avramouli, A.; Krokidis, M.G.; Exarchos, T.P.; Vlamos, P. In Silico Structural Analysis Predicting the Pathogenicity of PLP1 Mutations in Multiple Sclerosis. *Brain Sci.* **2022**, *13*, 42. [CrossRef] [PubMed]
7. Jiao, F.; Wang, M.; Sun, X.; Ju, Z.; Lu, J.; Wang, L.; Jiang, J.; Zuo, C. Based on Tau PET Radiomics Analysis for the Classification of Alzheimer's Disease and Mild Cognitive Impairment. *Brain Sci.* **2023**, *13*, 367. [CrossRef] [PubMed]
8. Jiang, J.; Zhang, J.; Li, C.; Yu, Z.; Yan, Z.; Jiang, J. Development of a Machine Learning Model to Discriminate Mild Cognitive Impairment Subjects from Normal Controls in Community Screening. *Brain Sci.* **2022**, *12*, 1149. [CrossRef] [PubMed]
9. Zhao, Y.; Zhang, J.; Chen, Y.; Jiang, J. A Novel Deep Learning Radiomics Model to Discriminate AD, MCI and NC: An Exploratory Study Based on Tau PET Scans from ADNI. *Brain Sci.* **2022**, *12*, 1067. [CrossRef] [PubMed]
10. Ju, Z.; Li, Z.; Lu, J.; Jiao, F.; Lin, H.; Bao, W.; Li, M.; Wu, P.; Guan, Y.; Zhao, Q.; et al. In Vivo Tau Burden Is Associated with Abnormal Brain Functional Connectivity in Alzheimer's Disease: A 18F-Florzolotau Study. *Brain Sci.* **2022**, *12*, 1355. [CrossRef]
11. Lee, C.C.; You, J.F.; Wang, Y.C.; Lan, S.W.; Wei, K.C.; Chen, K.T.; Huang, Y.C.; Wu, T.W.E.; Huang, A.P.H. Gross Total Resection Promotes Subsequent Recovery and Further Enhancement of Impaired Natural Killer Cell Activity in Glioblastoma Patients. *Brain Sci.* **2022**, *12*, 1144. [CrossRef] [PubMed]
12. Yi, T.; Zhan, A.; Wu, Y.; Li, Y.; Zheng, X.; Lin, D.; Lin, X.; Pan, Z.; Chen, R.; Parsons, M.; et al. Endovascular Treatment of ICAS Patients: Targeting Reperfusion Rather than Residual Stenosis. *Brain Sci.* **2022**, *12*, 966. [CrossRef] [PubMed]
13. Riso, V.; Nicoletti, T.F.; Rossi, S.; Vita, M.G.; Alessia, P.; Di Natale, D.; Silvestri, G. Neurological Erdheim–Chester Disease Manifesting with Subacute or Progressive Cerebellar Ataxia: Novel Case Series and Review of the Literature. *Brain Sci.* **2022**, *13*, 26. [CrossRef] [PubMed]
14. Moon, H.J.; Han, S. Perspective: Present and Future of Virtual Reality for Neurological Disorders. *Brain Sci.* **2022**, *12*, 1692. [CrossRef] [PubMed]

Disclaimer/Publisher's Note: The statements, opinions and data contained in all publications are solely those of the individual author(s) and contributor(s) and not of MDPI and/or the editor(s). MDPI and/or the editor(s) disclaim responsibility for any injury to people or property resulting from any ideas, methods, instructions or products referred to in the content.

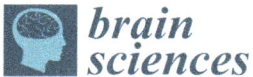

Article

Intermediate-Length GGC Repeat Expansion in NOTCH2NLC Was Identified in Chinese Patients with Amyotrophic Lateral Sclerosis

Mengxia Wan [1,2,†], Ji He [1,2,†], Junyan Huo [1,2], Can Sun [1,2], Yu Fu [1,2,*] and Dongsheng Fan [1,2,3,*]

1. Department of Neurology, Peking University Third Hospital, Beijing 100191, China
2. Beijing Municipal Key Laboratory of Biomarker and Translational Research in Neurodegenerative Diseases, Beijing 100191, China
3. Key Laboratory for Neuroscience, Ministry of Education/National Health Commission, Peking University, Beijing 100191, China
* Correspondence: lilac_fu@126.com (Y.F.); dsfan@sina.com (D.F.)
† These authors contributed equally to this work.

Abstract: GGC repeat expansions in the 5' untranslated region (5'UTR) of the Notch Homolog 2 N-terminal-like C gene (*NOTCH2NLC*) have been reported to be the genetic cause of neuronal intranuclear inclusion disease (NIID). However, whether they exist in other neurodegenerative disorders remains unclear. To determine whether there is a medium-length amplification of *NOTCH2NLC* in patients with amyotrophic lateral sclerosis (ALS), we screened 476 ALS patients and 210 healthy controls for the presence of a GGC repeat expansion in *NOTCH2NLC* by using repeat-primed polymerase chain reaction (RP-PCR) and fragment analysis. The repeat number in ALS patients was 16.11 ± 5.7 (range 7–46), whereas the repeat number in control subjects was 16.19 ± 3.79 (range 10–29). An intermediate-length GGC repeat expansion was observed in two ALS patients (numbers of repeats: 45, 46; normal repeat number ≤ 40) but not in the control group. The results suggested that the intermediate *NOTCH2NLC* GGC repeat expansion was associated with Chinese ALS patients, and further functional studies for intermediate-length variation are required to identify the mechanism.

Keywords: amyotrophic lateral sclerosis; *NOTCH2NLC*; intermediate-length repeats; nucleotide repeat expansion

1. Introduction

Recently, increasing numbers of repeat-expansion-related genes were identified as the causes of neurological disease [1]. Among them, a trinucleotide repeat (GGC) abnormal expansion in the 5′-untranslated region of the Notch Homolog 2 N-Terminal-Like C gene (*NOTCH2NLC*) in chromosome 1 attracted substantial attention and was reported as the cause of neuronal intranuclear inclusion disease (NIID) in Chinese and Japanese studies [2–4]. The *NOTCH2NLC* gene is one of the three paralogs of the NOTCH2 receptor, which plays a vital role in human cortex expansion [5]. NIID is a rare disease mainly involving nervous symptoms and is pathologically characterized by the presence of eosinophilic, p62- and ubiquitin-positive intranuclear inclusions in cells of the skin, peripheral and central nervous systems, and other visceral organs [6]. Furthermore, pathogenic expansion can be detected in a small proportion of patients with other neurological diseases such as dementia, Parkinson's syndrome, peripheral neuropathy, myopathy, leukoencephalopathy, and essential tremor.

In addition to finding new repeat-expansion-related genes and new links to various diseases, researchers have shown interest in the association between the length of repeat expansion and clinical types. Short repeats in *NOTCH2NLC* are associated with NIID Parkinson's disease dominant subtype (NIID-P), while the intermediate and long expansion is linked to NIID dementia dominant subtype (NIID-D) and myasthenic dominant subtype (NIID-M), respectively [7]. Intermediate-length repeat expansion refers to repeat sizes between normal and pathogenic ranges and has not previously received enough attention. Generally, the normal repeat size is less than 40 times in the general population, and the abnormal repeat size is more than 40 times. The pathogenic repeat expansion mutation is a repeat size exceeding 60 repeats, and the intermediate length is a repeat size between 40 and 60 repeats [7].

Amyotrophic lateral sclerosis (ALS) is a type of neurodegenerative disease that presents with insidious muscle weakness and atrophy caused by upper and lower motor neuron degeneration in the brain and spinal cord [8]. Motor neuron degeneration causes severe limb weakness, muscle fasciculations, disturbed speech, dysphagia, and death due to respiratory failure 3–5 years after disease onset. The etiology and risk factors for ALS remain unclear. Various genetic and environmental factors have been identified to contribute to the development of ALS [9]. To date, more than 40 genes have been identified to be associated with amyotrophic lateral sclerosis, and *SOD1*, *TARDBP*, *FUS*, and *C9ORF72* are the most common pathogenic genes in familial ALS (FALS) [10]. The intermediate-length (G4C2)n repeat expansion in *C9ORF72* and the CAG repeat expansion in *ATXN2* are associated with ALS and increase sporadic ALS(SALS) risk [11,12]. Identifying ALS-related genes can help to understand the disease's pathogenesis.

There are many similarities in clinical manifestations and pathological phenotypes between the NIID-M and ALS. For example, muscle weakness in limbs and ubiquitin- and p62-positive intranuclear inclusions can be found in NIID-M and ALS [6,13,14]. Furthermore, repeat-expansion-related genes play a vital role in ALS. Therefore, the association between the intermediate-length expansion of GGC in *NOTHCH2NLC* and ALS draws wide attention. In a study with 545 patients in mainland China, intermediate-length mutations were found [15]. However, in a study in Taiwan with 304 patients, no abnormal GGC expansion was found in ALS patients [16]. Owing to the clinical significance and current controversial results, further investigation is required to determine whether intermediate-length expansions specifically affect ALS.

In this study, we detected GGC repeat expansion in the *NOTCH2NLC* gene in a large cohort of Chinese ALS patients and investigated the relationship between *NOTCH2NLC* GGC repeat expansion and ALS. We found intermediate-length GGC repeat expansions in two ALS patients. The results suggested that the intermediate-length GGC repeat expansion in *NOTCH2NLC* was associated with ALS.

2. Methods

2.1. Subjects

The study included 476 Han Chinese ALS patients and 210 healthy controls from the Department of Neurology of Peking University Third Hospital between 2017 and 2020. All ALS cases met diagnostic criteria for ALS (the Escorial criteria [8]), with a diagnostic grade consistent with probable, suspected, or laboratory support-suspected diagnoses, and FALS patients with a family history were excluded. The patients had a negative gene screening test for *SOD1*, *TARDBP*, *FUS*, and *C9ORF72*. The control cohort was defined as people without possible neurodegenerative diseases, such as motor neuron disease, Alzheimer's disease, and Parkinson's disease, and a family history of the above diseases was excluded based on case records. The healthy control subjects were enlisted in the same area between 2017 and 2020. The age, sex, and race of the ALS group and the healthy control group were matched. The study was approved by the ethics committee of Peking University Third Hospital, and all participants signed informed consent forms. Study protocols were approved by the Ethics Committee review boards of Peking University Third Hospital. All human research in this study was conducted according to the Declaration of Helsinki.

2.2. Demographic and Clinical Data

Clinical data, including age, sex, history, family history, age of onset, and site of onset, were collected. Neurological examinations were administered by two neurologists experienced in treating ALS patients. The disease onset site was defined as bulbar onset or spinal onset. The Amyotrophic Lateral Sclerosis Functional Rating Scale (ALSFRS-R) was assessed to evaluate disease severity functional limitations in ALS patients. The Mini-Mental State Examination (MMSE) score, Edinburgh Cognitive and Behavior ALS Screen (ECAS), electromyogram (ECG), and cerebral fluid examinations were administered to some ALS patients. Demographic data in healthy controls, such as sex, age, and place of origin, were collected.

2.3. Blood Collection and DNA Extraction

Whole peripheral blood from participants was collected in ethylenediaminetetraacetic acid (EDTA) tubes. Genomic DNA was extracted using whole blood genomic DNA extraction kits (Aidlab Biotechnologies Co., Ltd, Beijing, China)DNA concentration and purity were assessed spectrophotometrically at 260 and 280 nm using a Nanodrop 2000. DNA was diluted to 20-100 ng/µL and used as a working solution.

2.4. Polymerase Chain Reaction Analysis

The *NOTCH2NLC* GGC repeat size was analyzed as previously described [3] but with small modifications. We used fragment analysis to identify the size of the fragment and repeat-primed PCR (RP-PCR) to identify whether it had abnormal expansions. For the fragment analysis, the PCR primer mix contained two primers, 0.3 µM *NOTCH2NLC*-F(5′-FAM- CATTTGCGCCTGTGCTTCGGAC-3′) and 0.3 µM *NOTCH2NLC*-R (5′-AGAGCGGCGCAGGGCGGGCATCTT-3′). For RP-PCR, the PCR primer mix contained three primers: 0.3 µM *NOTCH2NLC*-F(5′-FAM- GGCA TTTG CGCC TGTG CTTCGG ACCGT-3′), 0.3 µM M13-(GGC)4(GGA)2 R (5′- CAGGAAAC AGCT ATGA CCTC CTCC GCCG CCGCCGCC-3′, and 0.3 µM M13-linker-R(5′-CAGGAAACAGCTATGACC-3′). The PCR mix contained 0.25 U PrimeSTAR GXL DNA Polymerase, 1× PrimeSTAR GXL Buffer, 200 µM each dNTP Mixture (Takara Biomedical Technology (Beijing) Co., Ltd., Beijing, China), 5% dimethyl sulfoxide (sigma Aldrich (Shanghai) Trading Co., Ltd. Shanghai, China), 1 M betaine (Sigma-Aldrich), 0.3 µM each primer mix and 20–100 ng genomic DNA in a total reaction volume of 10 µL. For the two-primer PCR, the initial denaturation temperature was set at 98 °C for 10 min, then 30 cycles were initiated: 8 °C for 30 s, 58 °C for 1 min, and 68 °C for 2 min, followed by a final elongation step of 68 °C for 10 min. For the RP_PCR, the cycling conditions were set as follows: 16 cycles of 98 °C for 30 s, 72 °C for 15 s with a reduction of 0.5 °C per cycle, and 68 °C for 30 s, and 29 cycles of 98 °C for 30 s, 62 °C for 15 s and 68 °C for 30 s, followed by a final elongation step of 68 °C for 10 min. All PCR products were collected for capillary electrophoresis.

2.5. Capillary Electrophoresis

Electrophoresis was performed on a 3730xl DNA Analyzer (Applied Biosystems Inc, Foster City, USA) using the 500 LIZ dye Size Standard, and the data were analyzed by GeneMarker software. For the fragment analysis, the length of the highest signal peak of two-primer PCR product capillary electrophoresis in two alleles was used to calculate the repeat GGC size, and the larger one was used as the repeat size of the participants, as NIID is dominantly inherited. The calculation method was applied according to the results of first-generation sequencing in a standard patient and reference human genome hg38. Capillary electrophoresis of the RP-PCR product was used to identify the result, and a sawtooth tail pattern in the electropherogram was judged as abnormal repeat expansion.

2.6. Statistical Analysis

SPSS 22 was used for data processing. For measurement data, those with a normal distribution after inspection were expressed as the mean ± standard deviation ($x \pm s$). To explore the correlation between CSF protein level and GGC repeat size, Spearman's test was used. A two-tailed $p < 0.05$ was considered to demonstrate statistical significance.

3. Results

3.1. Clinical Data

A total of 476 patients were involved in this cohort, including 324 males and 152 females, and the control participants consisted of 120 males and 90 females. The mean age of ALS patients was 53.21 ± 11.66, while the age at enrollment for the control cohort was 52.58 ± 11.73. In total, 389 patients (81.7%) had initial spinal cord involvement, while 87 ALS patients (18.2%) had bulbar involvement initially. No patient had initial respiratory muscle involvement. A summary of the clinical features and demographic information of ALS and control participants is presented in Table 1.

Table 1. Demographic characteristics of ALS patients and healthy controls.

	ALS Patients	Healthy Controls
Total	476	210
Male	324 (68.07%)	120 (57.14%)
Female	152 (31.93%)	90 (42.86%)
Age at onset		
Mean ± SD	53.21 ± 11.66	52.58 ± 11.73 [a]
Site of onset		
Bulbar	87 (18.2%)	-
Spinal	389 (81.7%)	-

Abbreviations: SD: standard deviation. [a] Age at enrollment for the control cohort.

3.2. (GGC)n Expansion of NOTCH2NLC

By performing capillary electrophoresis of the two-primer PCR and repeated primer PCR product, we found that the repeat size was between 7 and 46 in the 476 ALS patients, and the mean number of repeats was 16.11 ± 5.7. Among them, 2 ALS cases (4.20%) had more than 40 repeats, and the repeats were 45 times and 46 times. RP-PCR revealed the sawtooth pattern, which identified abnormal repeat expansion (Figure 1).

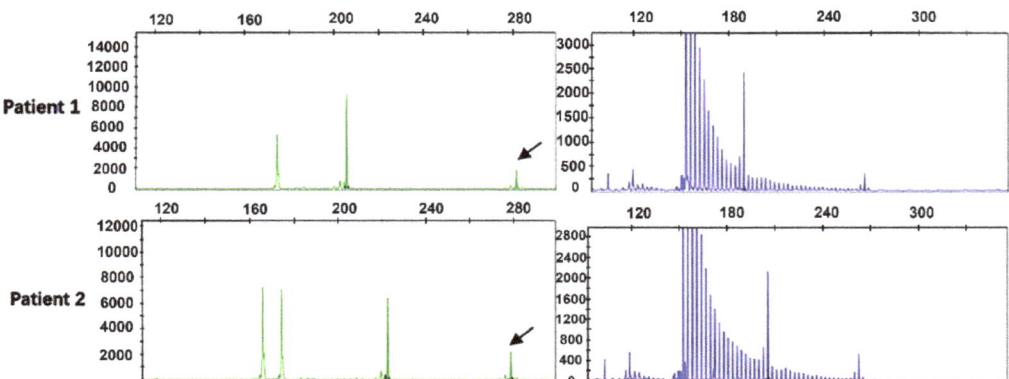

Figure 1. Fragment analysis (green) and repeat-primed PCR (blue) for two ALS patients harboring GGC intermediate-length repeat expansions. Fragment analysis showed the fragment size and the length of the highest signal peak (arrows). Repeat-primed PCR showed a sawtooth tail pattern of repeat expansion.

The repeat numbers in the controls were all less than 40 times, the repeat number was 10–29 in the controls, and the mean number of repeats was 16.19 ± 3.79. The distribution of the repeat sizes for the ALS patients and controls is shown in Figure 2.

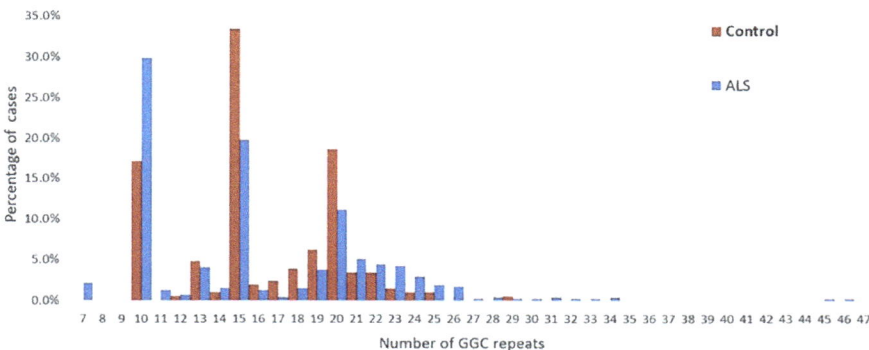

Figure 2. Distribution of the sizes of the NOTCH2NLC GGC repeats in 476 patients with ALS and 210 healthy controls.

3.3. Clinical Features

We summarized the clinical data of two identified ALS patients with intermediate-length GGC repeat, and the details are listed in Table 2.

Table 2. Clinical characteristics of amyotrophic lateral sclerosis patients with intermediate GGC repeat expansion.

Patient.No	Gender	Onset Age (y)	Site of Onset	Diagnosis Delay (mo)	Duration of Disease (mo)	ALS-FRS	NOTCH2NLC Repeat Size
1	male	50	Right lower limb	30	35	34	46
2	female	62	bilateral upper limbs	6	30	40	45

Abbreviations: ALS-FRS: ALS Functional Rating Scale.

Patient 1 was a 52-year-old male who carried 46 repeats. He initially presented with muscle weakness in the right foot at 50 years of age. Then, he showed muscle weakness in the four limbs and dysarthria gradually in the following two years. Neurological examination showed increased tendon reflexes in all extremities, and the Babinski sign, Hoffmann sign, abdominal reflex, and Maxillofacial reflex were all positive. Altogether, damage existed in the four upper motor units of the bulbar, cervical, thoracic and lumbar segments and three lower motor units of the bulbar, cervical, and lumbar segments. The ECAS score was 83, which is in the normal range. Brain magnetic resonance imaging (MRI) showed unspecific periventricular and subcortical white matter lesions (image unavailable). At that time, electromyography showed abundant and diffuse ongoing denervation (spontaneous potentials) and chronic reinnervation changes in the cervical, thoracic and lumbar segments. Sensory conduction studies showed compound muscle action potential (CMAP) reduction in both the ulnar and right median nerves. Pulmonary function indicated restrictive ventilatory dysfunction, the residual capacity ratio increased, and forced vital capacity (FVC) was 52%. Cerebrospinal fluid (CSF) examination showed elevated protein 338 mg/L, and oligoclonal bands were suspiciously positive both in the CSF and blood. He was clinically diagnosed with definite ALS in the third stage of KCSS and then died of respiratory failure 35 months after onset. Systemic examinations on tumor and immunological disease, including immunological index, tumor marker, and positron emission tomography computer tomography (PET-CT), were performed to exclude ALS mimics. Besides Riluzole, he had been treated with Intravenous Immunoglobulin Gamma (IVIG) because of his insistence. Nevertheless, IVIG did not improve his condition and prognosis.

Patient 2 was a female with 45 GGC. She complained of muscle weakness in both upper limbs at the age of 62. In the following two years, she suffered from muscle weakness in both lower limbs, dysarthria, and dysphagia. The patient was psychologically unstable in the past, regularly taking risperidone. In addition, she had transient cognitive impairment and urinary incontinence at the age of 61. Six months after onset, the physical examination showed damage in the three upper motor units of the bulbar, thoracic, and lumbar segments and one lower motor unit of the cervical segments. The cognitive function examination showed an ECAS score of 49 points and an MMSE score of 22 points, indicating cognitive impairment. Electromyography showed decreased amplitude in both upper extremity nerve motor conduction and the spontaneous potential of the bulbar and cervical segments. Brain MRI showed mild white matter lesions and lesions in the right parietal lobe, brain atrophy, and an enlarged ventricle (shown in Figure 3). According to history and imaging features, the lesion in the right parietal lobe was malacia due to cerebral infarction in the past.

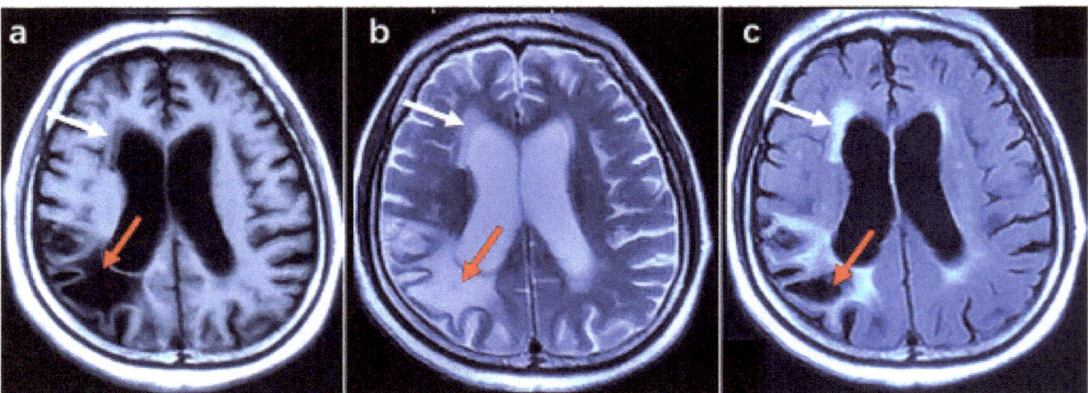

Figure 3. Brain MRI image in patient 2. (**a**) T1 weighted image, (**b**) T2 weighted image, (**c**) T2 Fluid-attenuated inversion recovery image. The red arrow shows malacia in the right parietal lobe, and the white arrow indicates a white matter lesion.

Thorough blood and CSF examinations were completed to exclude ALS mimics and other similar diseases. Unfortunately, diffusion-weighted image sequencing, which helps to identify NIID by exhibiting hyperintensities at the corticomedullary junction, was not performed as a result of the under-recognition of NIID at that time. CSF examination showed elevated protein 565.0 mg/L↑, and oligoclonal bands were suspiciously positive both in the CSF and blood, similar to patient 1. Memantine was administered to improve the patient's cognitive function. She was conclusively clinically diagnosed with ALS and then died of respiratory failure at 64 years of age, 30 months after the disease onset.

In summary, clinically, two patients presented with limbal muscle weakness and gradually developed more severe limb weakness, dysarthria, and dyspnea. Examination showed upper motor neuron signs in two patients (4 and 3 segments). Additionally, patient 2 presented with cognitive dysfunction, and two patients had mild white matter lesions, although we do not know if they were related to the intermediate-length expansion. No obvious abnormalities were identified in blood immunological function, inflammatory index, or serum tumor markers. No unusual findings were detected by electrocardiography or chest CT. Elevated protein was identified in the CSF, and suspicious oligoclonal bands were detected in the CSF and blood.

4. Discussion

In this study, we aimed to study the role of intermediate-length GGC repeat expansion in *NOTCH2NLC* in Chinese ALS patients. Therefore, we screened the *NOTCH2NLC* gene in 476 ALS patients and 210 controls and identified 2 intermediate-length GGC repeats 45 and 46 times in ALS patients and none in the control subjects, indicating that intermediate-length GGC repeat expansion is associated with ALS.

It has been shown that the GGC repeat expansion in *NOTCH2NLC* is associated with many neurologic disorders, such as Parkinson's disease, frontal temporal dementia, and essential tremor [17]. The GGC repeat size varies in NIID phenotypes and different neurological diseases [7]. The normal GGC range in *NOTCH2NLC* was 5–38 in healthy controls, while a repeat size > 60 indicated pathogenic GGC expansion [2]. More than 200 repetitions may increase susceptibility to NIID-M, and fewer than 100 repetitions may be associated with Parkinson's disease [7]. A total of 41-60 GGC repeats in *NOTCH2NLC* were defined as intermediate-length repeat expansions [18], which have been identified in many neurodegenerative diseases, such as Parkinson's disease, leukoencephalopathy, and Alzheimer's disease [2,18–22]. For Parkinson's disease, they found 11 patients with 41–52 repeats and 7 patients with 41–64 repeats in China and Singapore, respectively [18,19]. Fibroblasts from PD patients harboring intermediate-length repeat expansions revealed *NOTCH2NLC* upregulation and autophagic dysfunction, which suggested that medium-length repeat expansions in *NOTCH2NLC* were associated with PD [18]. Intermediate-length GGC repeats 42–58 and 42–47 times were found in patients with Alzheimer's disease and leukoencephalopathy, respectively [21,22].

For ALS, Yuan et al. [15] found that the repeat size ranged from 7 to 143 units and that GGC repeat expansion accounted for approximately 0.73% (4/545) of all ALS patients. They concluded that ALS was a specific phenotype of NIID or that GGC expansion in *NOTCH2NLC* was a modifiable factor for ALS. Similar to this study, intermediate GGC repeat expansion was also found in 2 ALS patients carrying 44 and 54 repeats. Nevertheless, no GGC repeat expansion was found in another study in Taiwan [16]. Our study provides evidence of the association between GGC repeat expansion and ALS. There are also other repeat-expansion-related genes linked to ALS risk. Ataxin-2 intermediate-length polyglutamine expansion is associated with increased ALS risk [12], and C9ORF72 intermediate-length repeat expansion is associated with corticobasal degeneration and ALS [11,23]. The significance of intermediate duplications, therefore, needs to be emphasized, and further studies in larger populations are needed to determine appropriate thresholds for pathogenic and normal duplications.

There are similarities in ALS patients with abnormal repeat expansion. There were more than three segments of the upper motor unit and lower motor unit dysfunction in these two patients with intermediate repeat expansion. The two patients both met the diagnostic criteria determined by the EI Escorial and Gold coast, and other diseases mimicking ALS were excluded [24]. We noted cognitive impairment in Patient 2 with 45 GGC repeats, similar to the two patients with 96 and 143 GGC repeat expansions in a previous study [15], who presented with memory impairment and behavioral impairment. In addition, a brain MRI showed mild white matter lesions in two patients, although the change was not specific. Mild leukoencephalopathy was previously found in patients with 54 GGC repeat expansions [15]. NIID patients mainly manifest cognitive dysfunction and leukoencephalopathy [6]. Another expansion disorder-related gene, C9ORF72, is the most common cause of familial frontotemporal dementia and ALS [25]. Although the current evidence is insufficient, these findings suggest that abnormal intermediate-length GGC repeats may be associated with cognitive impairment and white matter lesions in ALS.

The elevated CSF protein also attracted our attention. However, the literature shows that elevated CSF protein can be detected in both ALS and NIID [6]. Furthermore, we explored the correlation between CSF protein level and repeat number using the available CSF protein data in this ALS cohort. The results showed that the CSF protein level was not related to GGC repeat size using the Spearman correlation test. A previous study found that the CSF protein level determines a poor prognosis for spinal amyotrophic lateral sclerosis [26]. The cause and role of elevated CSF protein levels in ALS remain unclear, and the relationship between elevated CSF protein levels and intermediate-length expansion has not been studied. We can pay more attention to ALS patients with elevated CSF protein levels.

The overlap between NIID and ALS increased the difficulty of making a correct diagnosis. *NOTCH2NLC* repeat expansion was not found in the previous Taiwanese ALS cohort [16]. In addition, there are case reports that NIID may mimic the manifestations of ALS [27], and GGC repeat expansions in *NOTCH2NLC* (repeat size 248) lead to lower motor neuron syndrome [28]. Therefore, we need to be vigilant about whether the clinical diagnosis of ALS patients with abnormal or intermediate-length GGC expansion found by us was truly ALS. We can distinguish NIID-M from ALS by the following aspects, as Yuan et al. previously described [15]. First, ALS is often accompanied by damage in upper motor neurons, which leads to increased tendon reflexes and positive pathological signs, such as the Babinski sign and Hoffmann sign. Second, the prognosis of NIID-M is relatively better than that of ALS, and the disease duration is 16.6 and 3–5 years, respectively. Third, electromyography and nerve conduction studies provide useful information to make the correct diagnosis. The fibrillations and positive sharp-wave potentials cannot always exist in NIID-M patients, especially in the early stages of the disease. However, there are abundant and diffuse spontaneous potentials in ALS due to denervation. The performance in the nerve conduction study also differs in the NIID-M and ALS patients. Slow motor nerve conduction velocity (MCV) and sensory nerve conduction velocity (SCV) are more common in NIID-M. When considering the diagnosis of our two patients in this study, *NOTCH2NLC* can help us. The GGC repeat size in NIID is more than 60 times, and the repeat size in muscle weakness-dominant NIID is generally more than 200 times [2–4], while the GGC repeat size in the patients we reported is relatively small and cannot meet the repeat expansion criteria in NIID. In addition, the NIID case that mimics ALS has prominent lower motor neuron impairment, and upper motor unit impairment is not obvious [27], different from our patients, who have a three-regional upper and lower motor unit impairment. Therefore, enough evidence supports the ALS diagnosis.

The pathogenesis of GGC expansion in the *NOTCH2NLC* gene is currently unclear, and researchers have summarized the possible mechanisms, including (1) the toxicity of polyglycine-containing protein; (2) the toxicity of repeat RNA; (3) the GGC repeat size of *NOTCH2NLC*; (4) the size and types of trinucleotide interruption; and (5) the methylation status of *NOTCH2NLC* [7]. The current evidence mainly supports the formation of polyglycine-containing proteins. Recently, it has been certified that GGC trinucleotide repeats are translated into a polyglycine protein (N2NLCpolyG) through the upstream reading frame (uORF). N2NLCpolyG is rapidly degraded under normal conditions without GGC repeat expansion and does not produce aggregation, while the repeat expansion of GGC carried by the patient increases glycine numbers, which significantly enhances the stability and spontaneous aggregation of N2NLCpolyG, resulting in the formation of abnormal inclusion body-like protein aggregation [29,30]. Furthermore, N2NLCpolyG inclusions formed when GGC repeats expanded beyond 30, which may be one reason for the pathogenicity of medium-length expansions.

There were some limitations in our study. First, some important examinations were unavailable as the two patients passed away. Significant intensity signals in the DWI sequence in the corticomedullary junction and the inclusion body in the nervous system and skin were powerful cues for NIID diagnosis [6]. Nevertheless, we cannot obtain the two above examination results to provide more evidence to further distinguish ALS and NIID. Furthermore, the examination also helps to investigate the pathologic and imaging features in ALS with intermediate-length GGC expansions. Additionally, the number of control cases was 210 less than the ALS cohort, as the normal repeat size had been identified in other studies. Last, we did not perform experimental research to explore the mechanism of action of intermediate-length GGC repeats in *NOTCH2NLC* in ALS, and only two patients with intermediate-length GGC expansion were found, although the number of the cohort is not small regarding the incidence of ALS. In addition, it has also been reported that patients carrying intermediate repeat numbers are found in ALS patients [15], and in combination with our literature and reports from others, we believe that our speculation is justified. To identify the clinical features and mechanism, further studies are needed.

5. Conclusions

The present results suggest that intermediate-length GGC repeat expansion in *NOTCH2NLC* is associated with ALS. Larger cohorts in different geographic areas are required to further elucidate the characteristics of ALS with intermediate-length GGC, and basic experiments are needed to explore the mechanism of function.

Author Contributions: D.F. and Y.F. conceived and designed the study. M.W. performed the experiments. M.W. and J.H. (Ji He) collected and analyzed the data and wrote the paper. J.H. (Junyan Huo) and C.S. analyzed the genetic results. D.F. reviewed and edited the manuscript. All authors have read and agreed to the published version of the manuscript.

Funding: This study was funded by the National Natural Science Foundation of China (81873784, 82001347, and 82071426) and the Clinical Cohort Construction Program of Peking University Third Hospital, Grant/Award Number: BYSYDL2019002.

Institutional Review Board Statement: The study was approved by the ethics committees of Peking University Third Hospital (approval protocol number No. M2019388). All study protocols were in accordance with the Declaration of Helsinki. Informed consent was obtained from all subjects involved in the study.

Informed Consent Statement: Informed consent was obtained from all participants involved in the study.

Data Availability Statement: The data presented in this study are available upon request from the corresponding author. The data are not publicly available due to data management regulations in our hospital.

Conflicts of Interest: The authors report no conflict of interest.

References

1. Depienne, C.; Mandel, J.L. 30 years of repeat expansion disorders: What have we learned and what are the remaining challenges? *Am. J. Hum. Genet.* **2021**, *108*, 764–785. [CrossRef]
2. Tian, Y.; Wang, J.L.; Huang, W.; Zeng, S.; Jiao, B.; Liu, Z.; Chen, Z.; Li, Y.; Wang, Y.; Min, H.X.; et al. Expansion of Human-Specific GGC Repeat in Neuronal Intranuclear Inclusion Disease-Related Disorders. *Am. J. Hum. Genet.* **2019**, *105*, 166–176. [CrossRef]
3. Sone, J.; Mitsuhashi, S.; Fujita, A.; Mizuguchi, T.; Hamanaka, K.; Mori, K.; Koike, H.; Hashiguchi, A.; Takashima, H.; Sugiyama, H.; et al. Long-read sequencing identifies GGC repeat expansions in NOTCH2NLC associated with neuronal intranuclear inclusion disease. *Nat. Genet.* **2019**, *51*, 1215–1221. [CrossRef] [PubMed]
4. Ishiura, H.; Shibata, S.; Yoshimura, J.; Suzuki, Y.; Qu, W.; Doi, K.; Almansour, M.A.; Kikuchi, J.K.; Taira, M.; Mitsui, J.; et al. Noncoding CGG repeat expansions in neuronal intranuclear inclusion disease, oculopharyngodistal myopathy and an overlapping disease. *Nat. Genet.* **2019**, *51*, 1222–1232. [CrossRef] [PubMed]
5. Suzuki, I.K.; Gacquer, D.; Van Heurck, R.; Kumar, D.; Wojno, M.; Bilheu, A.; Herpoel, A.; Lambert, N.; Cheron, J.; Polleux, F.; et al. Human-Specific NOTCH2NL Genes Expand Cortical Neurogenesis through Delta/Notch Regulation. *Cell* **2018**, *173*, 1370–1384.e16. [CrossRef] [PubMed]
6. Sone, J.; Mori, K.; Inagaki, T.; Katsumata, R.; Takagi, S.; Yokoi, S.; Araki, K.; Kato, T.; Nakamura, T.; Koike, H.; et al. Clinicopathological features of adult-onset neuronal intranuclear inclusion disease. *Brain* **2016**, *139*, 3170–3186. [CrossRef]
7. Huang, X.R.; Tang, B.S.; Jin, P.; Guo, J.F. The Phenotypes and Mechanisms of NOTCH2NLC-Related GGC Repeat Expansion Disorders: A Comprehensive Review. *Mol. Neurobiol.* **2022**, *59*, 523–534. [CrossRef] [PubMed]
8. Brooks, B.R.; Miller, R.G.; Swash, M.; Munsat, T.L.; World Federation of Neurology Research Group on Motor Neuron Diseases. El Escorial revisited: Revised criteria for the diagnosis of amyotrophic lateral sclerosis. *Amyotroph Lateral Scler Other Mot. Neuron Disord* **2000**, *1*, 293–299. [CrossRef]
9. Feldman, E.L.; Goutman, S.A.; Petri, S.; Mazzini, L.; Savelieff, M.G.; Shaw, P.J.; Sobue, G. Amyotrophic lateral sclerosis. *Lancet* **2022**, *400*, 1363–1380. [CrossRef]
10. Chia, R.; Chio, A.; Traynor, B.J. Novel genes associated with amyotrophic lateral sclerosis: Diagnostic and clinical implications. *Lancet Neurol.* **2018**, *17*, 94–102. [CrossRef] [PubMed]
11. Iacoangeli, A.; Al Khleifat, A.; Jones, A.R.; Sproviero, W.; Shatunov, A.; Opie-Martin, S.; Alzheimer's Disease Neuroimaging, I.; Morrison, K.E.; Shaw, P.J.; Shaw, C.E.; et al. C9orf72 intermediate expansions of 24-30 repeats are associated with ALS. *Acta Neuropathol. Commun.* **2019**, *7*, 115. [CrossRef] [PubMed]

12. Elden, A.C.; Kim, H.J.; Hart, M.P.; Chen-Plotkin, A.S.; Johnson, B.S.; Fang, X.; Armakola, M.; Geser, F.; Greene, R.; Lu, M.M.; et al. Ataxin-2 intermediate-length polyglutamine expansions are associated with increased risk for ALS. *Nature* **2010**, *466*, 1069–1075. [CrossRef] [PubMed]
13. Takahashi-Fujigasaki, J.; Nakano, Y.; Uchino, A.; Murayama, S. Adult-onset neuronal intranuclear hyaline inclusion disease is not rare in older adults. *Geriatr. Gerontol. Int.* **2016**, *16* (Suppl. 1), 51–56. [CrossRef]
14. Saberi, S.; Stauffer, J.E.; Schulte, D.J.; Ravits, J. Neuropathology of Amyotrophic Lateral Sclerosis and Its Variants. *Neurol. Clin.* **2015**, *33*, 855–876. [CrossRef] [PubMed]
15. Yuan, Y.; Liu, Z.; Hou, X.; Li, W.; Ni, J.; Huang, L.; Hu, Y.; Liu, P.; Hou, X.; Xue, J.; et al. Identification of GGC repeat expansion in the NOTCH2NLC gene in amyotrophic lateral sclerosis. *Neurology* **2020**, *95*, e3394–e3405. [CrossRef]
16. Jih, K.Y.; Chou, Y.T.; Tsai, P.C.; Liao, Y.C.; Lee, Y.C. Analysis of NOTCH2NLC GGC repeat expansion in Taiwanese patients with amyotrophic lateral sclerosis. *Neurobiol. Aging* **2021**, *108*, 210–212. [CrossRef] [PubMed]
17. Cao, L.; Yan, Y.; Zhao, G. NOTCH2NLC-related repeat expansion disorders: An expanding group of neurodegenerative disorders. *Neurol. Sci.* **2021**, *42*, 4055–4062. [CrossRef]
18. Shi, C.H.; Fan, Y.; Yang, J.; Yuan, Y.P.; Shen, S.; Liu, F.; Mao, C.Y.; Liu, H.; Zhang, S.; Hu, Z.W.; et al. NOTCH2NLC Intermediate-Length Repeat Expansions Are Associated with Parkinson Disease. *Ann. Neurol.* **2021**, *89*, 182–187. [CrossRef]
19. Ma, D.; Tan, Y.J.; Ng, A.S.L.; Ong, H.L.; Sim, W.; Lim, W.K.; Teo, J.X.; Ng, E.Y.L.; Lim, E.C.; Lim, E.W.; et al. Association of NOTCH2NLC Repeat Expansions With Parkinson Disease. *JAMA Neurol.* **2020**, *77*, 1559–1563. [CrossRef]
20. Yau, W.Y.; Sullivan, R.; Rocca, C.; Cali, E.; Vandrovcova, J.; Wood, N.W.; Houlden, H. NOTCH2NLC Intermediate-Length Repeat Expansion and Parkinson's Disease in Patients of European Descent. *Ann. Neurol.* **2021**, *89*, 633–635. [CrossRef]
21. Jiao, B.; Zhou, L.; Zhou, Y.; Weng, L.; Liao, X.; Tian, Y.; Guo, L.; Liu, X.; Yuan, Z.; Xiao, X.; et al. Identification of expanded repeats in NOTCH2NLC in neurodegenerative dementias. *Neurobiol. Aging* **2020**, *89*, 142.e1–142.e7. [CrossRef] [PubMed]
22. Okubo, M.; Doi, H.; Fukai, R.; Fujita, A.; Mitsuhashi, S.; Hashiguchi, S.; Kishida, H.; Ueda, N.; Morihara, K.; Ogasawara, A.; et al. GGC Repeat Expansion of NOTCH2NLC in Adult Patients with Leukoencephalopathy. *Ann. Neurol.* **2019**, *86*, 962–968. [CrossRef] [PubMed]
23. Cali, C.P.; Patino, M.; Tai, Y.K.; Ho, W.Y.; McLean, C.A.; Morris, C.M.; Seeley, W.W.; Miller, B.L.; Gaig, C.; Vonsattel, J.P.G.; et al. C9orf72 intermediate repeats are associated with corticobasal degeneration, increased C9orf72 expression and disruption of autophagy. *Acta Neuropathol.* **2019**, *138*, 795–811. [CrossRef] [PubMed]
24. Shefner, J.M.; Al-Chalabi, A.; Baker, M.R.; Cui, L.Y.; de Carvalho, M.; Eisen, A.; Grosskreutz, J.; Hardiman, O.; Henderson, R.; Matamala, J.M.; et al. A proposal for new diagnostic criteria for ALS. *Clin. Neurophysiol.* **2020**, *131*, 1975–1978. [CrossRef] [PubMed]
25. DeJesus-Hernandez, M.; Mackenzie, I.R.; Boeve, B.F.; Boxer, A.L.; Baker, M.; Rutherford, N.J.; Nicholson, A.M.; Finch, N.A.; Flynn, H.; Adamson, J.; et al. Expanded GGGGCC hexanucleotide repeat in noncoding region of C9ORF72 causes chromosome 9p-linked FTD and ALS. *Neuron* **2011**, *72*, 245–256. [CrossRef] [PubMed]
26. Assialioui, A.; Dominguez, R.; Ferrer, I.; Andres-Benito, P.; Povedano, M. Elevated Cerebrospinal Fluid Proteins and Albumin Determine a Poor Prognosis for Spinal Amyotrophic Lateral Sclerosis. *Int. J. Mol. Sci.* **2022**, *23*, 11063. [CrossRef] [PubMed]
27. Fujita, A.; Ueno, T.; Miki, Y.; Arai, A.; Kurotaki, H.; Wakabayashi, K.; Tomiyama, M. Case report: Adult-onset neuronal intranuclear inclusion disease with an amyotrophic lateral sclerosis phenotype. *Front. Neurosci.* **2022**, *16*, 960680. [CrossRef] [PubMed]
28. Zhang, W.; Ma, J.; Shi, J.; Huang, S.; Zhao, R.; Pang, X.; Wang, J.; Guo, J.; Chang, X. GGC repeat expansions in NOTCH2NLC causing a phenotype of lower motor neuron syndrome. *J. Neurol.* **2022**, *269*, 4469–4477. [CrossRef]
29. Zhong, S.; Lian, Y.; Luo, W.; Luo, R.; Wu, X.; Ji, J.; Ji, Y.; Ding, J.; Wang, X. Upstream open reading frame with NOTCH2NLC GGC expansion generates polyglycine aggregates and disrupts nucleocytoplasmic transport: Implications for polyglycine diseases. *Acta Neuropathol.* **2021**, *142*, 1003–1023. [CrossRef]
30. Boivin, M.; Deng, J.; Pfister, V.; Grandgirard, E.; Oulad-Abdelghani, M.; Morlet, B.; Ruffenach, F.; Negroni, L.; Koebel, P.; Jacob, H.; et al. Translation of GGC repeat expansions into a toxic polyglycine protein in NIID defines a novel class of human genetic disorders: The polyG diseases. *Neuron* **2021**, *109*, 1825–1835.e5. [CrossRef]

Disclaimer/Publisher's Note: The statements, opinions and data contained in all publications are solely those of the individual author(s) and contributor(s) and not of MDPI and/or the editor(s). MDPI and/or the editor(s) disclaim responsibility for any injury to people or property resulting from any ideas, methods, instructions or products referred to in the content.

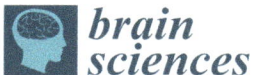

Case Report

Adult-Onset Neuronal Intranuclear Inclusion Disease with Mitochondrial Encephalomyopathy, Lactic Acidosis, and Stroke-Like (MELAS-like) Episode: A Case Report and Review of Literature

Qian Zhou [1], Meiqun Tian [2], Huan Yang [1] and Yue-Bei Luo [1,*]

[1] Department of Neurology, Xiangya Hospital, Central South University, Changsha 410008, China
[2] Department of Neurology, Hua Yuan People's Hospital, Jishou 416000, China
* Correspondence: yuebei507@126.com; Tel.: +86-073189753041

Abstract: Neuronal intranuclear inclusion disease (NIID) is a rare neurodegenerative disease with highly heterogeneous manifestations. Curvilinear hyperintensity along the corticomedullary junction on diffusion-weighted images (DWI) is a vital clue for diagnosing NIID. DWI hyperintensity tends to show an anterior-to-posterior propagation pattern as the disease progresses. The rare cases of its disappearance may lead to misdiagnosis. Here, we reported a NIID patient with mitochondrial encephalomyopathy, lactic acidosis and stroke-like (MELAS-like) episode, and reversible DWI hyperintensities. A review of the literature on NIID with MELAS-like episodes was conducted. A 69-year-old woman stated to our clinics for recurrent nausea/vomiting, mixed aphasia, altered mental status, and muscle weakness for 2 weeks. Neurological examination showed impaired mental attention and reaction capacity, miosis, mixed aphasia, decreased muscle strength in limbs, and reduced tendon reflex. Blood tests were unremarkable. The serological examination was positive for antibody against dipeptidyl-peptidase-like protein 6 (DPPX) (1:32). Brain magnetic resonance imaging (MRI) revealed hyperintensities in the left temporal occipitoparietal lobe on DWI and correspondingly elevated lactate peak in the identified restricted diffusion area on magnetic resonance spectroscopy, mimicking the image of MELAS. Skin biopsy and genetic testing confirmed the diagnosis of NIID. Pulse intravenous methylprednisolone and oral prednisolone were administered, ameliorating her condition with improved neuroimages. This case highlights the importance of distinguishing NIID and MELAS, and reversible DWI hyperintensities can be seen in NIID.

Keywords: neuronal intranuclear inclusion disease; NIID; mitochondrial dysfunction; MELAS; reversible DWI hyperintensities

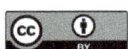

1. Introduction

Neuronal intranuclear inclusion disease (NIID) is a heterogeneous neurodegenerative disease, characterized by eosinophilic hyaline nuclear inclusions that are positive for ubiquitin and related proteins [1]. This disease can be sporadic or of an autosomal dominant inheritance. Recent research has identified the trinucleotide GGC repeat expansions in the 5′ untranslated region (5′ UTR) of the NOTCH2NLC gene in NIID [2,3].

Recently, Chinese researchers divided NIID into four subgroups based on the patients' initial and main clinical manifestations: dementia-dominant, movement disorder-dominant, muscle weakness-dominant, and paroxysmal symptom-dominant types [4]. Previous cases of paroxysmal symptoms have reported encephalitic episodes, stroke-like episodes, chronic headache, and mitochondrial encephalomyopathy, lactic acidosis, and stroke-like (MELAS-like) episode [4–7]. Due to its low incidence and high heterogeneity, diagnosis of NIID is often delayed or missed in clinical practice.

Fortunately, Sone in 2016 proposed diagnostic criteria for NIID, which mainly include positive skin biopsy, genetic examination, and typical magnetic resonance imaging (MRI)

findings [1]. Typical diffusion-weighted imaging (DWI) subcortical lace sign is considered an imaging marker for NIID with high specificity and sensitivity [8]. It tends to show an anterior-to-posterior propagation pattern. However, such lesions are more frequent in patients with dementia and paroxysmal symptoms types than in those with muscle weakness and movement disorder types [4]. It can also be absent in 10–20% of NIID patients, especially in the early disease course [8–10]. Reversible DWI hyperintensities have been reported in two cases in which hyperintense signals disappeared despite disease progression [11,12].

Reversible DWI hyperintensities can also present in MELAS syndrome, mostly caused by m.3243 A > G mutation in the MT-TL1 gene encoding the mitochondrial tRNA^{Leu} (UUR) [13]. It is a multi-organ disease with broad manifestations such as stroke-like episodes, dementia, epilepsy, lactic acidemia, myopathy, recurrent headaches, hearing impairment, diabetes, and short stature [13]. Patients tend to present stroke-like lesions inconsistent with vascular territory. These lesions with spontaneous reversibility are common in the posterior brain regions (i.e., the temporoparietal junction and the parietal and occipital lobes) [14]. Interestingly, patients with NIID can also present the above manifestations in MELAS syndrome.

Hitherto, MELAS-like episodes were only identified in two cases of NIID, among which one patient complained about chronic polyneuropathy and the other suffered recurrent migraine-attack [5,15]. Interestingly, reversible DWI hyperintensities were only seen in the case of polyneuropathy [5]. The other case presented progressed DWI hyperintensities [15]. Noticeably, several studies have also reported NIID patients with MELAS-like neuroimages, such as stroke-like lesions in the posterior brain regions (summarized in Table 1). However, the dynamics of these lesions are rarely observed.

Here, we report a sporadic NIID case mimicking MELAS episode, with detailed chronological neuroimaging. Different from the semeiology in previous cases, our patient presented recurrent nausea/vomiting, mixed aphasia, altered mental status, muscle weakness, and reversible DWI hyperintensities. A literature review is also conducted to summarize the characteristics of NIID patients with MELAS-like neuroimages, and thus better differentiate NIID and MELAS syndrome.

Table 1. The clinical characteristics of NIID patients with MELAS-like neuroimages.

References	Patient No.	Age, Sex	NOTCH2NLC GGC Repeats	Initial Symptoms	Clinical Manifestations	EEG	Nerve Conduction	Encephalitic Episode	FLAIR Brain Edema	T1W1+C Cortical Enhancement	DWI Hyperintense Lesions Cortical Lesions	DWI Hyperintense Lesions Corticomedullary Junction Lesions	Treatment
Our case	1	F/69	#	Amnesia	Headache; N/V; AMS; memory decline	LH diffuse SW	MD of motor nerve	+	+	-	+	+	Methylprednisolone
Xie [6]	2	F/51	118	Migraine	Headache; SD; urinary retention	N.A.	N.A.	+	+	+	+	+	Coenzyme Q10, riboflavin
Wang [7]	3	M/20	N.A.	Migraine	Headache; muscle weakness; SD; seizures; memory decline	N.A.	MD of motor nerve	+	+	-	+	+	Anti-seizure medications;
Okubo [16]	4	M/50	143	Tremor	Memory decline; tremor	N.A.	#	+	+	N.A.	+	+	N.A.
Ishihara [5]	5	F/47	*	Muscle weakness; SD	Headache; N/V; AMS	N.A.	#	+	+	+	+	-	Anti-seizure medications, edaravone, taurine
Liang [17]	6	F/56	115	Migraine	Headache; aphasia; fever; N/V; muscle weakness; SD; AMS; memory decline	RH diffuse SW	Normal	+	+	+	+	-	Methylprednisolone, dehydration
	7	F/35	98	migraine	Headache; N/V; muscle weakness; AMS; memory decline	BH sporadic SW	N.A.	+	+	+	+	+	Methylprednisolone, dehydration
	8	M/56	123	Dysuria; amnesia	Headache; bladder dysfunction; N/V; memory decline; AMS; SD	BH diffuse SW	AD of motor and sensory nerve	+	+	+	+	+	Methylprednisolone, dehydration
	9	F/61	110	Tremor	Headache; memory decline; bladder dysfunction; AMS; SD	BH diffuse SW and sporadic SSW	MD of sensory nerve	+	+	+	+	+	Methylprednisolone, dehydration
Liu [8]	10	F/48	136	N.A.	Headache; seizures; N/V	N.A.	N.A.	+	+	+	+	+	N.A.
	11	F/79	73	N.A.	AMS; seizures; aphasia; SD	N.A.	N.A.	+	+	+	+	+	N.A.
Mori [18]	12	F/61	N.A.	Parkinsonism	Headache; dysarthria; muscle weakness; AMS	N.A.	N.A.	+	+	+	+	+	Steroid therapy

No: number; F: female; M: male; N/V: nausea/vomiting; AMS: altered mental status; EEG: electroencephalograph; DWI: Diffusion weighted imaging; FLAIR: Fluid-attenuated inversion recovery images; T1W1+C: T1 weighted images with gadolinium enhancement; Rt: right; Lt: left; RH: right hemisphere; LH: left hemisphere; BH: bilateral hemisphere; SD: sensory disturbance; MD: myelin damage; AD: axonal damage; SW: slow waves; SSW: spine-slow integrated waves; N.A.: not available; -: negative; #: positive but without details; +: positive; *: (GGC)88(GGGA)1((GGC)4(GGA)2)9(GGC)4(GGA)1(GGC)3(GGA)2(GGC)2.

2. Materials and Methods

Clinical, imaging, and pathologic data were obtained from the patient's case files and clinical notes. Written informed consent was also obtained.

A review of the literature was conducted on PubMed and Web of Sciences (WOS), using the following research terms-" (NIID) OR (neuronal intranuclear inclusion disease)" and the features of MELAS neuroimage including" (MELAS) OR (occipital) OR (temporal) OR (cerebral edema) OR (leukoencephalopathy) OR (hyperperfusion) OR (cortical enhancement)". Fifties-six articles in PubMed and 64 articles in WOS have been identified. After deleting duplicates, 79 articles were scrutinized. All papers were screened by title, abstract, neuroimages, and main text. We selected papers in English reporting at least one case of NIID with MELAS-like images or episodes. Finally, eight articles have been found. For each case report/case series, the following information was attained: age, sex, NOTCH2NLC GGC repeats, initial symptoms, clinical manifestations, electroencephalograph (EEG); nerve conduction, episode, images, and treatment.

3. Results

The patient was a 69-year-old female farmer presenting with mild memory loss in the past two years, which did not hamper her social activity or farming. On 2 November 2021, she had a sudden visual hallucination, which resolved hours later. In the next few days, she developed headaches, recurrent vomiting, cognitive impairment, speech difficulty, and generalized weakness. She was admitted to the local hospital on November 6th, and her symptoms peaked three days after being hospitalized when she was completely bedridden. There were not any prodromal symptoms of fever. She had a ten-year history of diabetes and diabetic retinopathy, which were controlled by acarbose, gliclazide, and metformin.

Brain MRI in the local hospital one week after disease onset revealed symmetrical periventricular hyperintense signals on T2-weighted images, with diffuse brain atrophy and cerebral ventricle dilation (Figure 1). The lesions were unenhanced. Cerebrospinal fluid (CSF) examination indicated normal white blood cell count. Elevated protein (796 mg/L) and glucose (5.9 mmol/L) levels were observed in CSF. The testing of antibodies associated with autoimmune encephalitis and paraneoplastic syndrome revealed positive antibody against dipeptidyl-peptidase-like protein 6 (DPPX, titer 1:32) in the blood, while it was not found in CSF. Encephalitis was initially suspected. A follow-up MRI on November 11th found restricted diffusion in the left temporal occipitoparietal corticomedullary junction on DWI images and correspondingly elevated lactate peak on magnetic resonance spectroscopy (MRS), suggesting the possibility of MELAS. Pulse intravenous methylprednisolone (1 g) was given daily for three days and gradually tapered and replaced with oral prednisone. Her vomiting was alleviated, and muscle strength gradually improved. Cognitive disturbance was nevertheless persistent. She was referred to our hospital on 22 November.

Upon admission to our hospital, physical examination revealed normal vital signs. Neurological examination showed impaired mental attention and reaction capacity, miosis, mixed aphasia, decreased muscle strength in limbs generalized with MRC grading 4, and reduced tendon reflex. She could not cooperate with the examination of the muscle tone, brain nerve, ataxia, and sensory system. By then, she was unable to complete the mini-mental state examination (MMSE) scale and the Montreal cognitive assessment scale (MoCA).

Laboratory investigation revealed an elevated neutrophil percentage of 88.1 with a normal cell count. Blood glucose and glycated hemoglobin levels were elevated (11.43 mmol/L and 7.4%, respectively). Her serum creatine kinase, lactic acid, ketone, homocysteine, immunoglobulin, sex hormone, and cortisol level were all normal.

Electroencephalogram demonstrated diffuse slow waves (1.5–7 c/s) on the left hemisphere and limited sharp waves, especially on the frontotemporal lobe. Nerve conduction study was consistent with demyelinating polyneuropathy predominantly involving the motor nerves. The patient's bilateral median (left, 35.2 m/s and right, 42.3 m/s) and ulnar nerves (38.8 m/s on both sides) showed slow velocity. Motor conduction velocity of her bilateral tibial and peroneal nerves was also reduced to 30 m/s on average. Gynecological Sonography was normal. Repeated MRI on November 23rd showed restricted diffusion signals along the temporal occipitoparietal juxtacortex, and stenosis of M2 segments of the right middle cerebral artery and bilateral posterior cerebral arteries. Perfusion-weighted imaging (PWI) showed prominent hyperperfusion in the left occipitotemporal cortex (Figure 2). Faint DWI hyperintensity in the corticomedullary junction and high-intensity signals in the paravermis area were retrospectively recognized, suggesting the possibility of NIID.

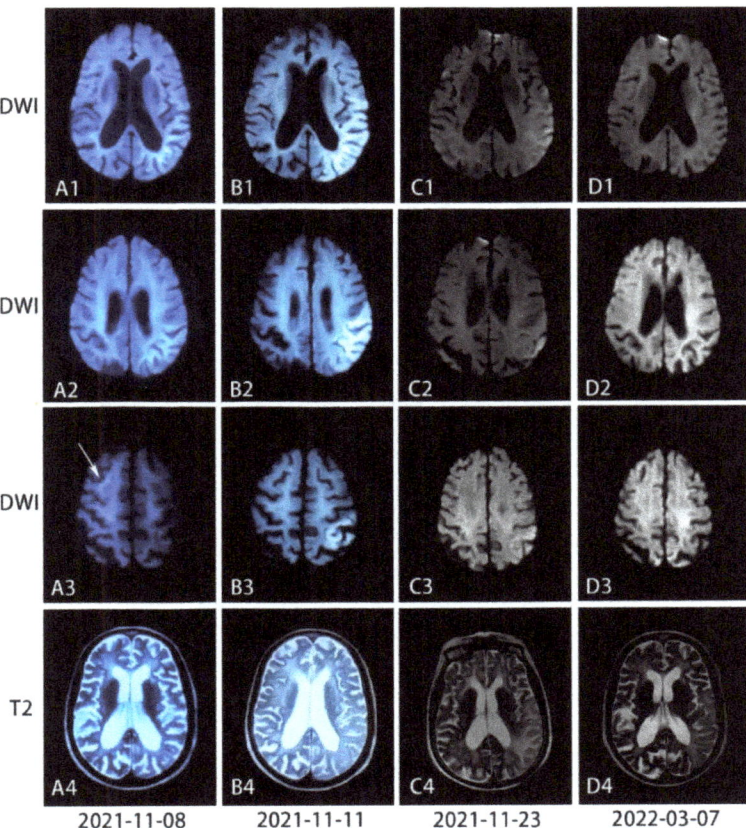

Figure 1. Chronological series of T2-weighted and diffusion-weighted images (DWI) images of the patient's brain. (**A**) Seven days after the disease onset when she had cognitive impairment, mixed aphasia, and muscle weakness, DWI showed curvilinear periventricular hyperintensity, while the T2-weighted image showed diffuse brain atrophy. (**B**) Two days after her symptoms exacerbated when she could be only bedridden, curvilinear lesions had transformed into confluent high-intensity lesions on DWI along the cortex in the temporal occipitoparietal lobe (in B1), where severe encephalopathy was also observed on the T2-weighted images. However, curvilinear hyperintensity in A3 disappeared. (**C**) Half a month after the peak and the treatment of pulse intravenous methylprednisolone, most high-intensity signals on DWI were eliminated but leukoencephalopathy and cortical edema on the T2-weighted scan were exacerbated. (**D**) Four months after the symptoms onset, high-intensity signals on DWI have vanished, while hyperintensity reduced with improved brain edema on T2-weighted images.

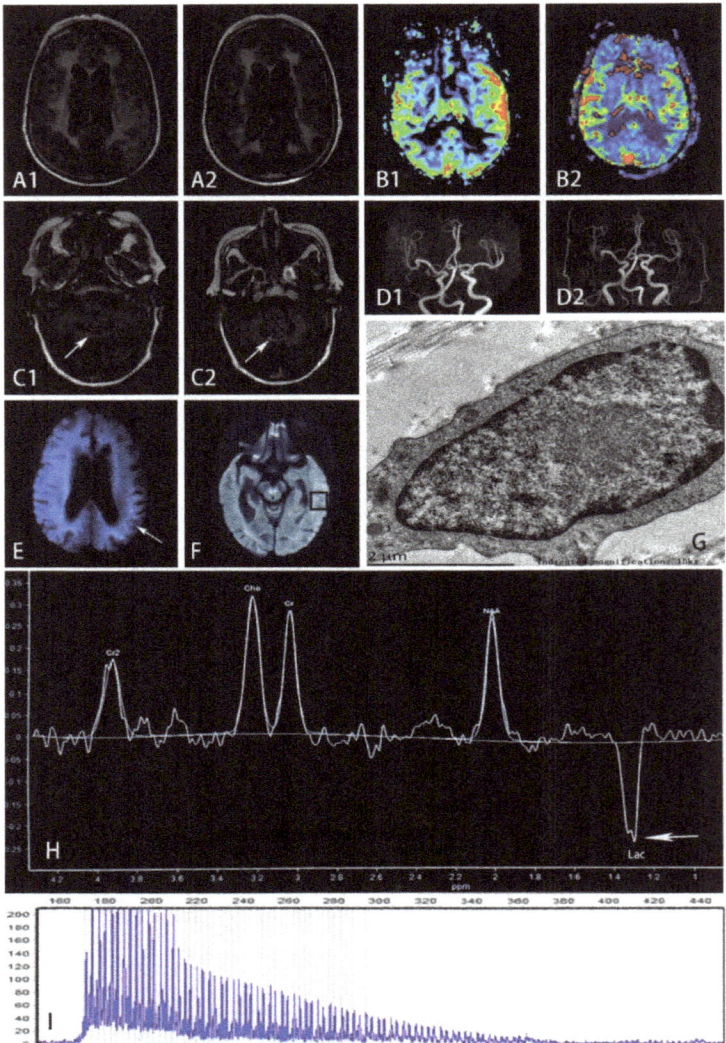

Figure 2. (**A**) FLAIR sequence on November 23rd (in A1) showed hyperintensity and edematous areas in the left temporal and occipital lobes, while such lesions improved 4 months later with reduced hyperintensity and less edema shown in A2. (**B**) PWI on November 23rd (in B1) showed prominent hyperperfusion in accordance with the lesion, but such phenomenon did not present after 4 months with symmetrical blood flow in bilateral temporal lobes shown in B2. (**C**) FLAIR sequence on November 23rd showed hyperintensity on the paravermis area (in C1), which remained the same after 4 months shown in C2. (**D**) MRA on November 23rd (in D1) showed the stenosis of M2 segments of the right middle cerebral artery, which was also presented after 4 months in D2. (**E**) The arrow refers to high-intensity areas in the corticomedullary junction on DWI on November 8th. (**G**) Electron microscopy of mechanocyte showed dense filamentous materials without limiting membrane. (**H**) MRS focusing on the temporal lesion (in (**F**)) showed the lactate peak appearance (shown by arrow). (**I**) RP-PCR showed GGC expansion in the patient. (FLAIR, fluid-attenuated inversion recovery; PWI, perfusion-weighted image; DWI, diffusion-weighted image; MRA, magnetic resonance angiography; MRS, magnetic resonance spectroscopy; RP-PCR, repeat-primed PCR; Lac, lactate).

Skin biopsy samples were obtained 10 cm above the patient's ankle. Electron microscopy showed round-shaped intranuclear inclusions, composed of dense filamentous materials without membrane structure. However, eosinophilic ubiquitin-positive and p62-positive intranuclear inclusions were not found. Repeat-primed PCR confirmed the diagnosis of adult-onset NIID (>66 repeats of GGC in the 5'UTR of the NOTCH2NLC gene). Her family history was unremarkable. Our patient and her brother were entrusted to their relatives since childhood, and they soon lost contact with their parents. Her brother with diabetes did not suffer from migraine, stroke, or deafness. Her offspring are healthy. No DNAs of other family members were available.

During hospitalization, oral prednisolone was gradually tapered. Her cognitive deficiency was gradually alleviated, and she could briefly communicate when she was discharged. After returning home, the patient had recurrent vomiting for a week but resolved spontaneously.

On follow-up three months after discharge, she had pupils of diameters within normal range. She was ambulant and alert. MMSE score was 18 and MOCA was 8, indicating moderate cognitive impairment. A follow-up brain MRI revealed the DWI high intensity of the occipitotemporal lobe had largely resolved, while brain atrophy progressed.

4. Discussion

Here we report a patient with NIID presenting with an acute MELAS-like episode and neuroimaging. She had insidious onset of cognitive impairment, and the disease was exacerbated by a MELAS-like episode. Brain imaging showed diffuse white matter hyperintensity, brain atrophy, and a largely reversible parietooccipital lesion. Despite the positive anti-DPPX antibody, the diagnosis of autoimmune encephalitis was dismissed as the clinical picture did not conform to the phenotype associated with anti-DPPX encephalitis [19]. Lactate peak on MRS and hyperperfusion in the lesion have been reported in both MELAS and NIID [5]. Nevertheless, no muscle volume reduction or myogenic changes on electromyography (EMG) have been detected. The late onset age and lack of any family history of muscle weakness or stroke-like episodes made the diagnosis of mitochondrial disease very unlikely. The faint corticomedullary lesion on DWI highly suggestive of NIID resolved as the MELAS-like episode ended, but hyperintensity of the paravermis area persisted. Such neuroimages suggested the possibility of NIID.

Corticomedullary hyperintensity on DWI is a strong image marker for NIID with an anterior-to-posterior propagation pattern [8]. Previous literature has also identified high DWI signals in the corpus callosum, severe leukoencephalopathy involving the corpus callosum, middle cerebellar peduncle, paravermis area, and cortical edema with gadolinium enhancement as useful clues. Cerebral atrophy and lateral ventricle enlargement were often observed in the late stages [4].

Interestingly, Sone reported that 21% of adult-onset NIIDs experienced a subacute encephalitic episode with characteristic symptoms including fever, headache, vomiting, and loss of consciousness [1]. NIID patients with encephalopathy tend to have cortical hyperintensity distributed in the parietal-occipital lobes, in contrast to curvilinear DWI hyperintensity preferentially located in the frontoparietal region [8]. These lesions are not distributed following vascular supply [8]. One-fifth of encephalitis-like NIID cases could have FLAIR hyperintense lesions with edematous changes and contrast enhancement [8]. Okubo reported a NIID patient with focal hypoperfusion at the acute stage of encephalitis-like episode and rebound hyperperfusion several days later [16]. Ataka and Ishihara reported hyperperfusion in the abnormal cortices [5,20]. The increased peak of lactate point on MRS can also be observed in NIID [5].

Similar to the encephalopathy of NIID, cortical swelling and hyperperfusion can also present in MELAS. Therefore, it can easily be confused with the neuroimaging of MELAS.

To summarize the characteristics of NIID with MELAS-like neuroimaging, we reviewed the literature and found another 11 cases with MELAS-like neuroimages (Table 1). All patients with MELAS-like neuroimages experienced encephalitis-like episodes. A third of the patients used to have migraine. They tend to present headaches (83.3%), altered mental status (66.7%), memory decline (58.3%), and nausea/vomiting (50.0%) during an episode. All patients who received examination of electroencephalograph presented slow waves. Myelin damages (60%) were more frequent than axonal damages (20%). All patients have brain edema and cortical lesions. Cortical enhancement and DWI corticomedullary hyperintensities have been shown in most cases.

Interestingly, the aforementioned manifestations can also be present in MELAS syndrome, except corticomedullary hyperintensities on DWI. Thus, curvilinear hyperintensity along the corticomedullary junction on DWI is a useful tool for differential diagnosis.

Unlike previous cases with cortical enhancement, which is purposed as a brain image marker for the differential diagnosis between MELAS and NIID with MELAS-like episodes, our patient did not present such enhancement. In fact, such enhancement can also be seen in MELAS due to hyperemia or luxury perfusion [13]. Furthermore, our case showed the disappearance of DWI hyperintensities as the episode ended, reversed to the common idea that this signal would not fade away once appeared. Skin biopsy, with a high degree of consistency with NOTCH2NLC gene detection, can reveal eosinophilic intranuclear inclusions, immunopositive for ubiquitin and p62, composed of fibrous materials without membranous structures [21]. However, fibrous materials without membranes were identified in mechanocyte nucleus under electron microscope, while immunofluorescence staining was negative in our patient.

Eosinophilic intranuclear inclusions are valuable diagnostic clues. It can be detected more than 10 years before the onset of the symptoms and found in morphologically intact neurons without obvious neuronal loss. Previous literature demonstrated the positive rate of electron microscopy was lower than that of immunostaining due to limitations in the sampling and observation scope [21,22]. However, it is exactly opposite in our patient. Cao also reported two patients with negative pathological findings [22]. Though the underlying mechanism is unclear, the loss of p62/SQSTM1 has been reportedly associated with accelerating aging and age-related pathologies [23]. Moreover, eosinophilic ubiquitin-positive inclusions can also be observed in fragile X-associated tremor/ataxia syndrome (FXTAS) in neurons, glial cells, and somatic cells, though no skin pathological or electron microscopic findings of intranuclear inclusions have been identified in FXTAS [1]. NIID and FXTAS shared similar clinical manifestations. Thus, it is difficult to distinguish NIID from FXTAS with only the histopathological findings. For this reason, gene tests should be performed. NIID is diagnosed based on abnormal repeat expansion of GGC (>65 repeats) within the 5' UTR of the NOTCH2NLC gene [4].

Though curvilinear hyperintensity along the corticomedullary junction is a useful tool to differentiate MELAS and NIID with MELAS episode, it can be absent or reversible in rare cases. Some researchers observed such hyperintensities were absent at the onset but presented in the corticomedullary junction area 6 years later, and ultimately disappeared 8 years after onset in a NIID patient [24]. Researchers suspected the pathological spongiotic changes in subcortical white matter proximal to U-fibers may be the culprit of DWI hyperintensities [11,25]. Subsequent edema withdrawal, neuronal loss, and gliosis may account for the disappearance of DWI hyperintensities and the widening of cerebral sulci [11]. Moreover, patients with MELAS can present spontaneous reversibility in both neurological symptoms and neuroimages [14]. Once such curvilinear hyperintensities disappear, it is easily misdiagnosed.

To distinguish between NIID with MELAS-like episodes and MELAS syndrome, we should consider the following conditions. For clinical features, most patients with confirmed MELAS have a maternal genetic history and present between 2 and 40 years of age, mostly before age 15. They had systemic symptoms including loss of hearing, growth failure, and diabetes, which are distinguished from phenotypes of NIID [14]. For auxiliary examination, an electrophysiological study might aid the differentiation. Nerve conduction studies of MELAS patients typically show an axonal or mixed axonal and demyelinating neuropathy, similar to NIID in which demyelination is more frequent than axonal damage [1,13]. EMGs of MELAS patients tend to show myogenic changes. In addition to corticomedullary hyperintensities on DWI, basal ganglia calcification and iron deposition can be frequently seen in MELAS, while they can also be presented in the elders [13]. High intensity in the paravermis area might be a useful indicator to distinguish NIID as it is rarely reported in other patients with leukoencephalopathies [4]. Muscle and skin biopsy, as well as gene testing aid the confirmative diagnosis.

Bearing many commonalities in clinical and imaging characteristics, NIID is suspected to have similar pathogenesis to MELAS. Noticeably, previous researchers also identified abnormal mitochondrial inclusions in patients with NIID [26]. Yu et al., recently developed a fly model of CGG repeat expansion in NOTCH2NLC, recapitulated key pathological and clinical features of NIID, and characterized the mitochondrial dysfunction in these model organisms, human samples, and cellular models [27]. Here, we proposed three possible mechanisms linking NIID to mitochondrial dysfunction. First, large CGG repeats may stall the replication fork leading to a double-strand break and chromosome fragility, which further affects mitochondrial homeostasis [28]. Second, expanded CGG repeats may sequester specific RNA binding proteins resulting in altered splicing and decreased miRNA biogenesis. Decreased expression of miRNAs leads to their altered translocation to the mitochondria [29]. Lastly, polyG forms intranuclear inclusion may affect the transport of miRNA/mRNAs and nuclear-encoded mitochondrial proteins to the mitochondria. These effects can finally result in bioenergetic crisis, elevated reactive oxygen species, and cell death [29]. The secondary mitochondrial abnormalities may at least partly explain the overlapping presentations and neuroimages of NIID and MELAS.

5. Conclusions

This case report portrays a patient with NIID who presented MELAS-like episode and reversible DWI hyperintensities. Patients with MELAS-like neuroimaging tend to present headaches, altered mental status, memory decline, and nausea/vomiting during an episode. DWI curvilinear hyperintensity could aid the differentiation between NIID and MELAS, but its disappearance might lead to misdiagnosis. To distinguish between NIID with MELAS-like episodes and MELAS syndrome, we should consider some special clinical manifestations, EMG, and neuroimaging. High DWI signals in the corpus callosum and severe leukoencephalopathy involving the corpus callosum, middle cerebellar peduncle, and paravermis area can help the diagnosis of NIID. Muscle and skin biopsy, as well as gene testing aid the confirmative diagnosis.

Author Contributions: Conceptualization: Y.-B.L. Drafting the manuscript: Q.Z., M.T., H.Y. and Y.-B.L. Editing and final draft: Q.Z. and Y.-B.L. All authors have read and agreed to the published version of the manuscript.

Funding: This research received no external funding.

Institutional Review Board Statement: The study was conducted in accordance with the Declaration of Helsinki, and approved by the Ethics Committee of the Xiangya Hospital of Central South University. (IRB{S} NO.2022020582).

Informed Consent Statement: Written informed consent has been obtained from the patient to publish this paper.

Conflicts of Interest: The authors declare no conflict of interest.

References

1. Sone, J.; Mori, K.; Inagaki, T.; Katsumata, R.; Takagi, S.; Yokoi, S.; Araki, K.; Kato, T.; Nakamura, T.; Koike, H.; et al. Clinicopathological features of adult-onset neuronal intranuclear inclusion disease. *Brain* **2016**, *139*, 3170–3186. [CrossRef] [PubMed]
2. Sone, J.; Mitsuhashi, S.; Fujita, A.; Mizuguchi, T.; Hamanaka, K.; Mori, K.; Koike, H.; Hashiguchi, A.; Takashima, H.; Sugiyama, H.; et al. Long-read sequencing identifies GGC repeat expansions in NOTCH2NLC associated with neuronal intranuclear inclusion disease. *Nat. Genet.* **2019**, *51*, 1215–1221. [CrossRef] [PubMed]

3. Deng, J.; Gu, M.; Miao, Y.; Yao, S.; Zhu, M.; Fang, P.; Yu, X.; Li, P.; Su, Y.; Huang, J.; et al. Long-read sequencing identified repeat expansions in the 5′UTR of the NOTCH2NLC gene from Chinese patients with neuronal intranuclear inclusion disease. *J. Med. Genet.* **2019**, *56*, 758–764. [CrossRef] [PubMed]
4. Tian, Y.; Zhou, L.; Gao, J.; Jiao, B.; Zhang, S.; Xiao, Q.; Xue, J.; Wang, Y.; Liang, H.; Liu, Y.; et al. Clinical features of NOTCH2NLC-related neuronal intranuclear inclusion disease. *J. Neurol. Neurosurg. Psychiatry* **2022**. [CrossRef]
5. Ishihara, T.; Okamoto, T.; Saida, K.; Saitoh, Y.; Oda, S.; Sano, T.; Yoshida, T.; Morita, Y.; Fujita, A.; Fukuda, H.; et al. Neuronal intranuclear inclusion disease presenting with an MELAS-like episode in chronic polyneuropathy. *Neurol. Genet.* **2020**, *6*, e531. [CrossRef] [PubMed]
6. Xie, F.; Hu, X.; Liu, P.; Zhang, D. A Case Report of Neuronal Intranuclear Inclusion Disease Presenting With Recurrent Migraine-Like Attacks and Cerebral Edema: A Mimicker of MELAS. *Front. Neurol.* **2022**, *13*, 837844. [CrossRef] [PubMed]
7. Wang, R.; Nie, X.; Xu, S.; Zhang, M.; Dong, Z.; Yu, S. Interrelated Pathogenesis? Neuronal Intranuclear Inclusion Disease Combining With Hemiplegic Migraine. *Headache* **2020**, *60*, 382–395. [CrossRef] [PubMed]
8. Liu, Y.H.; Chou, Y.T.; Chang, F.P.; Lee, W.J.; Guo, Y.C.; Chou, C.T.; Huang, H.C.; Mizuguchi, T.; Chou, C.C.; Yu, H.Y.; et al. Neuronal intranuclear inclusion disease in patients with adult-onset non-vascular leukoencephalopathy. *Brain* **2022**, *145*, 3010–3021. [CrossRef]
9. Tamura, A.; Fujino, Y.; Sone, J.; Shiga, K. Temporal Changes in Brain Magnetic Resonance Imaging Findings over 16 Years in a Patient with Neuronal Intranuclear Inclusion Disease. *Intern. Med.* **2021**, *60*, 2483–2486. [CrossRef]
10. Okamura, S.; Takahashi, M.; Abe, K.; Inaba, A.; Sone, J.; Orimo, S. A case of neuronal intranuclear inclusion disease with recurrent vomiting and without apparent DWI abnormality for the first seven years. *Heliyon* **2020**, *6*, e04675. [CrossRef]
11. Kawarabayashi, T.; Nakamura, T.; Seino, Y.; Hirohata, M.; Mori, F.; Wakabayashi, K.; Ono, S.; Harigaya, Y.; Shoji, M. Disappearance of MRI imaging signals in a patient with neuronal intranuclear inclusion disease. *J. Neurol. Sci.* **2018**, *388*, 1–3. [CrossRef] [PubMed]
12. Chen, L.; Wu, L.; Li, S.; Huang, Q.; Xiong, J.; Hong, D.; Zeng, X. A long time radiological follow-up of neuronal intranuclear inclusion disease: Two case reports. *Medicine* **2018**, *97*, e13544. [CrossRef] [PubMed]
13. El-Hattab, A.W.; Adesina, A.M.; Jones, J.; Scaglia, F. MELAS syndrome: Clinical manifestations, pathogenesis, and treatment options. *Mol. Genet. Metab.* **2015**, *116*, 4–12. [CrossRef]
14. Tetsuka, S.; Ogawa, T.; Hashimoto, R.; Kato, H. Clinical features, pathogenesis, and management of stroke-like episodes due to MELAS. *Metab. Brain Dis.* **2021**, *36*, 2181–2193. [CrossRef] [PubMed]
15. Zeng, W.G.; Liao, W.M.; Hu, J.; Chen, S.F.; Wang, Z. Mitochondrial encephalomyopathy, lactic acidosis, and stroke-like episodes (MELAS) syndrome mimicking herpes simplex encephalitis: A case report. *Radiol. Case Rep.* **2022**, *17*, 2428–2431. [CrossRef] [PubMed]
16. Okubo, M.; Doi, H.; Fukai, R.; Fujita, A.; Mitsuhashi, S.; Hashiguchi, S.; Kishida, H.; Ueda, N.; Morihara, K.; Ogasawara, A.; et al. GGC Repeat Expansion of NOTCH2NLC in Adult Patients with Leukoencephalopathy. *Ann. Neurol.* **2019**, *86*, 962–968. [CrossRef]
17. Liang, H.; Wang, B.; Li, Q.; Deng, J.; Wang, L.; Wang, H.; Li, X.; Zhu, M.; Cai, Y.; Wang, Z.; et al. Clinical and pathological features in adult-onset NIID patients with cortical enhancement. *J. Neurol.* **2020**, *267*, 3187–3198. [CrossRef]
18. Mori, K.; Yagishita, A.; Funata, N.; Yamada, R.; Takaki, Y.; Miura, Y. Imaging findings and pathological correlations of subacute encephalopathy with neuronal intranuclear inclusion disease-Case report. *Radiol. Case Rep.* **2022**, *17*, 4481–4486. [CrossRef]
19. Piepgras, J.; Höltje, M.; Michel, K.; Li, Q.; Otto, C.; Drenckhahn, C.; Probst, C.; Schemann, M.; Jarius, S.; Stöcker, W.; et al. Anti-DPPX encephalitis: Pathogenic effects of antibodies on gut and brain neurons. *Neurology* **2015**, *85*, 890–897. [CrossRef]
20. Ataka, T.; Kimura, N.; Matsubara, E. Temporal Changes in Brain Perfusion in Neuronal Intranuclear Inclusion Disease. *Intern. Med.* **2021**, *60*, 941–944. [CrossRef]
21. Pang, J.; Yang, J.; Yuan, Y.; Gao, Y.; Shi, C.; Fan, S.; Xu, Y. The Value of NOTCH2NLC Gene Detection and Skin Biopsy in the Diagnosis of Neuronal Intranuclear Inclusion Disease. *Front. Neurol.* **2021**, *12*, 624321. [CrossRef] [PubMed]
22. Cao, Y.; Wu, J.; Yue, Y.; Zhang, C.; Liu, S.; Zhong, P.; Wang, S.; Huang, X.; Deng, W.; Pan, J.; et al. Expanding the clinical spectrum of adult-onset neuronal intranuclear inclusion disease. *Acta Neurol. Belg.* **2022**, *122*, 647–658. [CrossRef] [PubMed]
23. Bitto, A.; Lerner, C.A.; Nacarelli, T.; Crowe, E.; Torres, C.; Sell, C. P62/SQSTM1 at the interface of aging, autophagy, and disease. *Age* **2014**, *36*, 9626. [CrossRef] [PubMed]
24. Wang, H.; Feng, F.; Liu, J.; Deng, J.; Bai, J.; Zhang, W.; Wang, L.; Xu, B.; Huang, X. Sporadic adult-onset neuronal intranuclear inclusion disease without high-intensity signal on DWI and T2WI: A case report. *BMC Neurol.* **2022**, *22*, 150. [CrossRef] [PubMed]
25. Yokoi, S.; Yasui, K.; Hasegawa, Y.; Niwa, K.; Noguchi, Y.; Tsuzuki, T.; Mimuro, M.; Sone, J.; Watanabe, H.; Katsuno, M.; et al. Pathological background of subcortical hyperintensities on diffusion-weighted images in a case of neuronal intranuclear inclusion disease. *Clin. Neuropathol.* **2016**, *35*, 375–380. [CrossRef]
26. Morimoto, S.; Hatsuta, H.; Komiya, T.; Kanemaru, K.; Tokumaru, A.M.; Murayama, S. Simultaneous skin-nerve-muscle biopsy and abnormal mitochondrial inclusions in intranuclear hyaline inclusion body disease. *J. Neurol. Sci.* **2017**, *372*, 447–449. [CrossRef]
27. Yu, J.; Liufu, T.; Zheng, Y.; Xu, J.; Meng, L.; Zhang, W.; Yuan, Y.; Hong, D.; Charlet-Berguerand, N.; Wang, Z.; et al. CGG repeat expansion in NOTCH2NLC causes mitochondrial dysfunction and progressive neurodegeneration in Drosophila model. *Proc. Natl. Acad. Sci. USA* **2022**, *119*, e2208649119. [CrossRef]

28. Liufu, T.; Zheng, Y.; Yu, J.; Yuan, Y.; Wang, Z.; Deng, J.; Hong, D. The polyG diseases: A new disease entity. *Acta Neuropathol. Commun.* **2022**, *10*, 79. [CrossRef]
29. Gohel, D.; Berguerand, N.C.; Tassone, F.; Singh, R. The emerging molecular mechanisms for mitochondrial dysfunctions in FXTAS. *Biochim. Biophys. Acta Mol. Basis Dis.* **2020**, *1866*, 165918. [CrossRef]

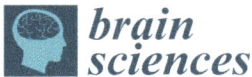

Article

In Silico Structural Analysis Predicting the Pathogenicity of PLP1 Mutations in Multiple Sclerosis

Antigoni Avramouli, Marios G. Krokidis *, Themis P. Exarchos and Panagiotis Vlamos

Bioinformatics and Human Electrophysiology Laboratory, Department of Informatics, Ionian University, 491 00 Corfu, Greece
* Correspondence: mkrokidis@ionio.gr

Abstract: The X chromosome gene *PLP1* encodes myelin proteolipid protein (PLP), the most prevalent protein in the myelin sheath surrounding the central nervous system. X-linked dysmyelinating disorders such as Pelizaeus–Merzbacher disease (PMD) or spastic paraplegia type 2 (SPG2) are typically caused by point mutations in *PLP1*. Nevertheless, numerous case reports have shown individuals with *PLP1* missense point mutations which also presented clinical symptoms and indications that were consistent with the diagnostic criteria of multiple sclerosis (MS), a disabling disease of the brain and spinal cord with no current cure. Computational structural biology methods were used to assess the impact of these mutations on the stability and flexibility of PLP structure in order to determine the role of *PLP1* mutations in MS pathogenicity. The analysis showed that most of the variants can alter the functionality of the protein structure such as R137W variants which results in loss of helix and H140Y which alters the ordered protein interface. In silico genomic methods were also performed to predict the significance of these mutations associated with impairments in protein functionality and could suggest a better definition for therapeutic strategies and clinical application in MS patients.

Keywords: myelin proteolipid protein; protein structure prediction; functional analysis; multiple sclerosis

1. Introduction

Myelination is an important process of the CNS that provides electrical insulation to axons and facilitates the transmission of nerve impulses. This protective layer is formed by Schwann cells in the peripheral nervous system, while oligodendrocytes form the sheath in the CNS [1]. The myelin sheath is a multi-layered membrane composed of proteins and lipids (approximately 30% and 70%, respectively). The lipid composition contains high amounts of cholesterol, phospholipids and glycolipids [2]. PLP is one of the major myelin proteins which, together with the DM20 isoform resulting from alternative splicing, constitutes 50% of the total protein. PLP plays a crucial role in the formation and maintenance of proper myelin structure and stability in the CNS [3]. It is a transmembrane and hydrophobic protein, with 48% of its sequence being non-polar or aromatic amino acids including 14 cysteine residues, which either undergo post-translational modifications and bind to fatty acids or are involved in intramolecular disulfide bonds. It has been observed that patients suffering from MS have an increased population of T-cells specific for PLP peptides and increased levels of anti- $PLP_{181-230}$ specific antibodies were found in serum levels compared to healthy individuals and patients with other neurological diseases [4]. Human and rodent PLP share several epitopes that are recognized by T cells [5]. Other main counterparts are myelin basic protein (MBP), which constitutes 30% of the total myelin protein in the CNS, myelin oligodendrocyte glycoprotein (MOG) and myelin-associated glycoprotein (MAG) [6–8]. Smaller percentage is occupied by alpha-beta crystallin, a small heat shock protein [9].

Multiple sclerosis (MS) is a chronic demyelinating inflammatory condition affecting the human central nervous system (CNS) [10]. It is unclear whether MS begins in the periphery,

Citation: Avramouli, A.; Krokidis, M.G.; Exarchos, T.P.; Vlamos, P. In Silico Structural Analysis Predicting the Pathogenicity of PLP1 Mutations in Multiple Sclerosis. *Brain Sci.* **2023**, *13*, 42. https://doi.org/10.3390/brainsci13010042

Academic Editors: Woon-Man Kung and Dina Nur Anggraini Ningrum

Received: 2 December 2022
Revised: 19 December 2022
Accepted: 20 December 2022
Published: 24 December 2022

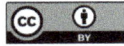

Copyright: © 2022 by the authors. Licensee MDPI, Basel, Switzerland. This article is an open access article distributed under the terms and conditions of the Creative Commons Attribution (CC BY) license (https://creativecommons.org/licenses/by/4.0/).

through activation of immune cells that then penetrate the CNS and cause damage, or within the CNS through primary damage to myelin or oligodendrocyte [11,12]. This could be the result of mutations in molecules encoding essential myelin or oligodendrocyte components, even though genome-wide association studies have not indicated substantial associations with any of these in MS [13]. However, the possibility that mutations in genes encoding these components are present in some proportions of MS patients remains under consideration. To that end, missense mutations in *PLP1* gene have been described in patients with clinical symptoms consistent with an MS diagnosis, such as an amino acid substitution at residue 31 of PLP (L31V) in a female patient with primary progressive MS [14]. Mutations can largely affect protein functionality, hence analysis of potential alterations in protein tertiary structure can reveal new evidence for their effect on phenotype. A novel mutation in *PLP1* exon 2 that changed leucine to arginine (L31R) was reported in a mother and her son through sequencing of the *PLP1* gene [15]. In a recent study, a mother and daughter with a preliminary diagnosis of primary progressive MS carried a nonsense mutation at codon 210 T > G [16]. Moreover, a L31P mutation was also associated with severe PMD [17]. The transmembrane portion of PLP1/DM20 proteins could be disrupted by both mutations, affecting intracellular trafficking. Neuroinflammation and axonal neurodegeneration was also reported in mice carrying the R137W and L31R mutations by one year of age [18].

The structure and function of the native protein may be significantly altered by missense mutations, particularly those in the coding area that modify the amino acid configuration. In order to determine the impact of each nonsynonymous single nucleotide polymorphism (nsSNP) in a related protein, it is common practice to functionally compare mutant proteins with their wild-type counterparts associated with specific traits in vitro [19]. However, the experimental design for each mutational modification is time- and labor-intensive. Thus, it is feasible and cost-effective to perform data mining for mutational analysis and functional prediction on protein properties using computational methods [20]. The three-dimensional (3D) structure of a protein has a pivotal role in protein's functional characterization. There are many efficient structural biology algorithms for predicting tertiary protein structures based on their amino acid sequences. Therefore, considering the role of the *PLP1* gene in spontaneous myelin and axonal damage, we retrieved all mutations in the *PLP1* gene related to MS. Using in silico structural and functional analyses, this study aimed to describe potential disease-associated variants of the *PLP1* gene.

2. Materials and Methods

A variety of different computational approaches was used to screen out the functional effects of the variants in the *PLP1* gene related to MS. The methodology we followed is divided into four distinct levels, including (i) primary data collection, (ii) creation of the 3D protein structures, (iii) 3D protein structure comparison process (iv) variant functional analysis. A baseline method raised from pure bioinformatics approaches was utilized as a benchmark for validation.

2.1. Summary of Variants

Five variants of *PLP1* gene and specifically the association of three of them with multiple sclerosis were analyzed in our study. The transcript sequence and the protein encoded by the *PLP1* gene were retrieved from the Ensembl database [21]. Then, the UniProt ID for the amino acid (P60201–MYPR_HUMAN) was obtained from UniProt Protein Database.

2.2. In Silico Methods for Predicting Mutation Significance

dbNSFP database was used for functional prediction and annotation of potential non-synonymous single-nucleotide variants (nsSNVs). The current version of this high-performance variant annotation tool can be queried to extract prediction scores from 38 algorithms [22,23]. dbNSFP also provides conservation scores and supplementary data, such as allele frequencies, functional gene descriptions, gene expression and gene interaction data, etc. MutPred2 machine learning-based approach was implemented to predict the pathogenicity of amino acid substitutions and their molecular mechanisms [24].

Further computational tools such as ANNOVAR (https://annovar.openbioinformatics.org/en/latest/, accessed on 16 September 2022), KGGSeq (http://pmglab.top/kggseq/, accessed on 16 September 2022), VarSome (https://varsome.com, accessed on 16 September 2022), UCSC Genome Browser's Variant Annotation Integrator (http://genome.ucsc.edu/cgi-bin/hgVai, accessed on 19 September 2022), Ensembl Variant Effect Predictor (http://www.ensembl.org/info/docs/tools/vep/index.html, accessed on 20 September 2022), SnpSift (https://pcingola.github.io/SnpEff/, accessed on 20 September 2022) and HGMD (https://www.hgmd.cf.ac.uk/ac/index.php, accessed on 22 September 2022) were used to strengthen the analysis, and the outcomes were validated using each platform separately. The algorithms utilized in this study are publicly accessible for all academic, non-commercial uses.

2.3. Protein Stability Correlation Analysis

The correlation between mutations and protein stability was analyzed based on a lesser decrease in free energy (ΔG or dG). Alterations in protein stability are determined by differences in free energy ($\Delta\Delta G$ or ddG) between wild-type and mutant proteins [25]. The DynaMut server was used to assess the effect of a single point mutation on protein stability, conformation, and flexibility, and to visualize protein dynamics [26]. DynaMut provides more accurate (p-value < 0.001) assessments of the effects of single mutations on protein stability than other well-established methods. In addition, the DynaMut server defines $\Delta\Delta G \geq 0$ as stabilizing and $\Delta\Delta G < 0$ for comparison purposes. In addition, Site Directed Mutator (SDM) server was used to estimate the change in protein stability following mutation [27].

2.4. Analysis of Protein Structural Conformation and Conservation

ConSurf server (http://consurf.tau.ac.il/, accessed on 7 October 2022) was utilized to identify highly conserved functional areas of the PLP1 gene-encoded protein [28].

2.5. Prediction of the Secondary Structure

Using the PSIPRED server (http://bioinf.cs.ucl.ac.uk/psipred/, accessed on 10 October 2022), the secondary structure of PLP1 was predicted [29]. It is based on a two-stage neural network with position-specific scoring matrices derived from PSI-BLAST to predict the available secondary structures of a protein.

2.6. Homology Modeling

SWISS-MODEL was utilized to determine the three-dimensional structure of PLP1. The CAMEO system determines the precision of the generated model. SWISS-MODEL is based on evolutionary information and searches a high-throughput template library (SMTL) for the optimum sequence–template alignment to construct the model [30]. Phyre-2 server was used to predict the homology-based three-dimensional structure of the query amino acid sequence [31]. I-TASSER was selected for protein structure prediction and structure-based function annotation [32–34]. Initially, structural templates from the PDB are discovered using LOMETS, a multithreaded algorithm. With the templates as guides, full-length atomic models are then constructed using simulations of fragment assembly iterations. The 3D models are re-run through the BioLiP database of protein functions to gain insight into the target's function. C-I-TASSER, an enhanced version of I-TASSER designed to accurately predict protein structures and functions was used to generate inter-residue contact maps beginning with a query sequence [34]. The structural templates of the PDB are derived by the multithreaded method LOMETS, and their full-length atomic models are constructed using contact maps and replica exchange Monte Carlo simulations. Finally, COFACTOR uses the structural model to deduce the protein's biological functions.

C-I-TASSER produces significantly more accurate models than I-TASSER in large-scale benchmark tests.

2.7. Mutated Structure Prediction

Once the mutations were identified, the construction protein-based structures in PDB format were followed. I-TASSER and DynaMut servers were used to perform the transformation of the amino acid sequences to 3D protein models. Then, for each model, structural alignment was carried out and the structural similarity score was calculated. The TM-align and TM-score algorithms were selected for the alignment and the similarity score calculation, respectively [35].

2.8. Protein Three-Dimensional Model Verification

Three-dimensional structures were validated using Ramachandran plot analysis (http://molprobity.biochem.duke.edu, accessed on 19 October 2022). It provides the number of residues that are located in the allowed, favored, and outlier regions. If a significant fraction of residues resides in the allowed and favored region, it is projected that the model is accurate [36].

3. Results

3.1. PLP1 Variants Associated with MS

PLP consists of 276 amino acid residues and four hydrophobic transmembrane domains, and its expression is restricted to oligodendrocyte cells. The area of the *PLP1* gene that encodes residue 31 appears to be a hotspot for mutation, since it has been described in MS patients (L31R and L31V mutation) [14]. In cases of severe PMD, the L31P mutation has also been documented [14]. The idea of mutation hotspots in *PLP1* has been previously characterized in PMD patients, and numerous mutations have been detected in a number of amino acids [37]. R137W mutation has also been described in MS patients, while the H140Y one was selected because it is the closest known mutation to residue 137 [14]. Detailed information about the variants analyzed in the current study is shown in Table 1.

Table 1. PLP1 variants. This mutation was selected as the closest mutation to residue 137 known for *PLP1*.

Location	Codon Change	Amino Acid Position	Amino Acid Alteration	Description [1]
X:103785668	CTG/GTG	31	L/V	MS- like disease mutation
X:103785669	CTG/CCG	31	L/P	Severe PMD mutation
X:103785669	CTG/CGG	31	L/R	MS- like disease mutation
X 103786682	CGG/TGG	137	R/W	MS- like disease mutation
X 103786691	CAT/TAT	140	H/Y	Mild SPG2 mutation

[1] MS: multiple sclerosis; PLP: myelin proteolipid protein; PMD: Pelizaeus–Merzbacher disease; SPG2: spastic paraplegia type 2.

3.2. Variant Functional Analysis

There are numerous assessment strategies for missense variants and recent databases include results from a variety of techniques to assist the evaluation of the impact of variations predicted to modify the peptide sequence of a gene. Herein, using dbNSFP, we investigated the functional consequences of missense SNPs, including whether they are normal, disease-causing, or effective by chance. As Table 2 shows, functional analysis revealed that R137W, L31P, L31V, L31R are damaging from the most prediction tools with a high score, while the results for H140Y were different across the different methods.

Table 2. Functional analysis of PLP variants using dbNSFP.

Variant	L31P	L31V	L31R	R137W	H140Y	Range (Low to Damaging)
Polyphen2_HDIV_score	0.999	0.997	0.999	0.999	0.015	0.03061 to 0.91137
LRT_converted_rankscore	0.8433	0.8433	0.8433	0.4496	0.53742	0.00162 to 0.8433
MutationTaster_score	1	0.999999	1	0.627105	0.281663	0 to 1
MutationTaster_converted_rankscore	0.81001	0.58761	0.81001	0.81001	0.81001	0.08979 to 0.81001
MutationAssessor_score	2.71	2.36	2.71	1.24	0.69	−5.17 to 6.49
MetaLR_score	0.9794	0.9771	0.9794	0.9547	0.9047	0 to 1
MetaRNN_score	0.988245	0.946438	0.98141	0.892939	0.962404	0 to 1
MutPred_score	0.932	0.813	0.887	0.663	0.779	0 to 1
DEOGEN2_score	0.994664	0.910984	0.994756	0.707527	0.697598	0 to 1
ClinPred_score	0.996376	0.982601	0.997494	0.958003	0.509568	0 to 1

We strengthened our analysis using further computational tools such as ANNOVAR, KGGSeq and VarSome and the outcomes were validated using each platform separately.

The results of MutPred2 demonstrated that these variants may alter the function of protein structures (Table S1). MutPred2 provides a general score which represents the average of all neural network scores based on a ranked list of specific molecular alterations potentially affecting the phenotype, and therefore, this number indicates the probability that the amino acid substitution could be harmful. A score threshold of 0.50, if considered as a probability, could reveal pathogenicity. However, a threshold of 0.68 results in a false positive rate (fpr) of 10%, whereas a threshold of 0.80 results in an fpr of 5%. In our case, L31P (score 0.973), L31V (score 0.854), and L31R (score 0.972) mutations may result in an altered transmembrane protein (Table S1). The R137W variant (score 0.684) may lead to a loss of helix, whereas the H140Y variant (score 0.556) may result in a changed ordered interface or transmembrane protein.

3.3. Conformational Analysis and Alteration of Protein Stability upon Amino Acid Substitution

DynaMut predicts the change in stability by calculating the changes in unfolding Gibbs free energy ($\Delta\Delta G$), as summarized in Table 3. For comparison, $\Delta\Delta G$ predictions based on protein structure were also displayed including dinstinct approaches and assumptions. Parallel analysis was performed using Site Directed Mutator (SDM) computational methods to verify the molecular effect of the five variants (Table S2). Three of them (L31V, L31P L31R) revealed a diminution in stability by increasing the molecular flexibility of the wild-type proteins (Tables 3 and S2). On the contrary, H140Y variant enhanced the stability of the PLP1 protein. R137W variant revealed conflicting results. DynaMut demonstrated that the amino acid changes in R137W decrease stability, while SDM exhibited elevated stability (Table S2). ENCoM analysis was executed to calculate the vibrational entropy difference (ΔS) between wild-type and mutant structures as well as to explore protein conformational space and the effect of mutations on protein function and stability. As Figure 1 illustrates, the mutation causes a change in the vibrational entropy of the amino acid.

Table 3. Conformational Analysis of Protein's Stability Change upon Amino Acid Substitution.

Variant	$\Delta\Delta G$ (kcal/mol)	Outcome	$\Delta\Delta S$VibENCoM (kcal.mol^{-1}.K^{-1})	Outcome [1]
L31V	−0.133	Destabilizing	0.083	Increase
L31P	−1.011	Destabilizing	0.413	Increase
L31R	−0.256	Destabilizing	0.231	Increase
R137W	−0.400	Destabilizing	0.111	Increase
H140Y	0.519	Stabilizing	−0.063	Decrease

[1] Molecule flexibility.

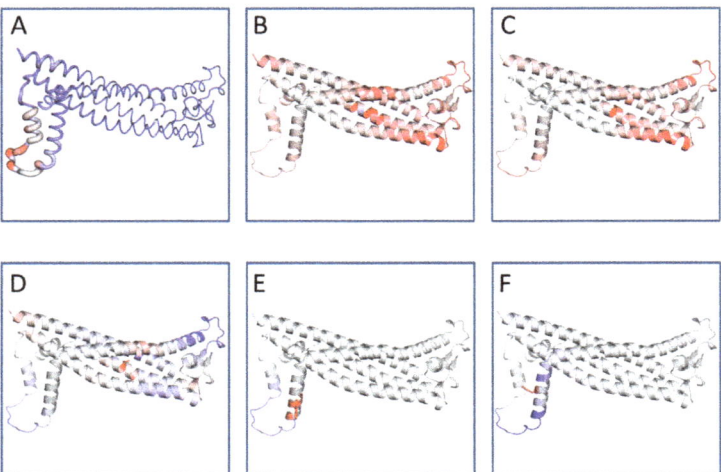

Figure 1. Protein flexible conformation based on the Vibrational Entropy difference (ΔΔS) between wild-type and mutant structures on the structure of PLP1. A visual representation of the chain in which the mutation occurs is also mapped. Amino acids colored according to the vibrational entropy change upon mutation. Blue represents a rigidification of the structure and red represents a gain in flexibility. (**A**) Normal PLP1; (**B**) L31P mutant; (**C**) L31R mutant; (**D**) L31V mutant; (**E**) R137W mutant; (**F**) H140Y mutant. The image is illustrated by DynaMut. The positions of the point mutations are 31, 137 and 140. Abbreviations: L is leucine; P is proline; R is arginine; V is valine; W is tryptophan; H is histidine; Y is tyrosine.

3.4. Analysis of the Structural Conformation and Conservation of PLP1

According to ConSurf analysis, the variants located at position 31 (L31V, L31P, and L31R) were found in a highly conserved region with a conservation score of 9 (Figure 2). Based on this indication, we can estimate that these nsSNPs play a functional role on the protein conformation. On the contrary, R137 and H140 displayed a conservation score of 1 (Figure S1).

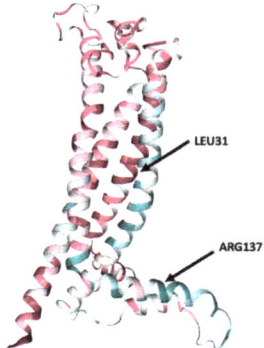

Figure 2. ConSurf analysis of conserved functional areas of the structural model of PLP1 gene-encoded protein. Amino acid at positions 31 (leucine) and 137 (arginine) are highlighted. Leucine in position 31 is a highly conserved region. Conservation score is presented in Figure S1.

3.5. PLP1 Protein Secondary Structure Prediction

The alpha helix, beta sheet distribution and coils for PLP1 were calculated according to PSIPRED protein structure prediction server. Among the exposed secondary structures, the highest in percentage was alpha helix (65%) followed by coils (30%) and no beta-sheet (0.0%) (Figure S2).

3.6. Prediction Software Benchmarking and Creation of Tertiary Protein Structures

Using four distinct homology modeling techniques, the three-dimensional (3D) structures of the PLP1-encoded protein were reconstructed. Since only 3% of residues 45–53 is represented on the protein data bank (https://www.ebi.ac.uk/pdbe/pdbe-kb/, accessed on 10 October 2022), there was no known crystal data of this protein of the appropriate length. Once the mutations were identified, the next step was to construct protein-based structures to represent these variants. Since the 3D protein feature view was not determined through experimental methodologies, established computational tools and databases such as Uniprot (UniProt Consortium, London, UK, 2015), Swiss-Model, Phyre-2, I-TASSER, C-I-Tasser, PDBeFold and Dynamut were evaluated for predicting the mutated structures and calculated the effect of these domain mutations on the 3D protein structure.

Based on the Hidden Markov approach, the Phyre-2 server was implemented to predict the homology-based three-dimensional structure of the query amino acid sequence. It incorporates five phases to construct a model: (1) collection of homologous sequences, (2) screening of fold library, (3) modeling of loops, (4) ab initio folding simulation Poing for multiple template modeling, and (5) placement of side chains [31]. Tertiary protein structures were formed based on the available structure prediction tools. Out of an extensive benchmarking of the structural predictive tools, we selected to retrieve the PLP1 target structure from the AlphaFold database. Comparison results revealed that AlphaFold reached the highest accuracy between predicted and experimental structure. In Figure 3, the visualization of the predicted 3D model of PLP1 protein is presented as performed by AlphaFold, Phyre-2, I-TASSER and C-I-Tasser, respectively, as these servers exhibited the highest accuracy in predicting the experimental structure. The model–template alignment by Swiss Model retrieved structures that did not include amino acids involved in the present outcomes.

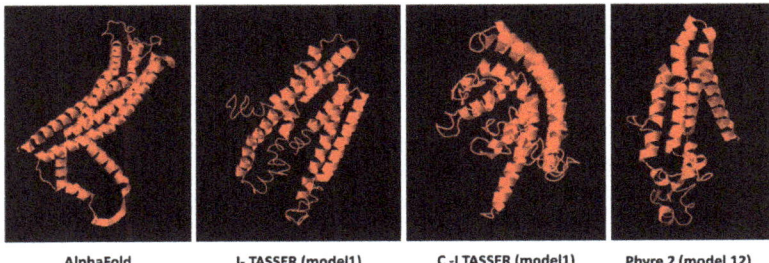

Figure 3. Protein structure prediction models of PLP1 calculated by different computational methodologies. AlphaFold model presented high confidence for the residue of the protein at position 31 (pLDDT > 90), but limited confidence for the PLP1 residue at position 137 (pLDDT < 50). Model 1 showed the highest C- score (−3.95) in I-TASSER and C-I-Tasser (−3.89) servers. Phyre2 model 12 with a confidence of 16.98% was the only one that included the residues analyzed in this study.

3.7. Variant Tertiary Protein Structures

The next step in our pipeline was to construct the structures for these mutations using I-TASSER and DynaMut [26]. The DynaMut provides a comprehensive evaluation and visualization of protein mobility and flexibility using two independent, well-established normal mode approaches to analyze protein dynamics by sampling conformations. In parallel, assessment of the effect of mutations on protein dynamics and stability due to changes in vibrational entropy can be executed. The server combines graph-based signatures with normal mode dynamics to predict the influence of a selected mutation on protein stability. The predicted models were compared against the corresponding AphaFold structure through the TM-align algorithm and a benchmarking of the structural predictive tools was accomplished. Comparative results revealed that DynaMut reached the highest accuracy between the predicted and experimental structure and was also used to verify the impact of mutations on protein conformation, flexibility and stability as well as to visualize protein dynamics. The TM-score is the metric that will lead to the selection of the ideal approach for producing the potential tertiary structures of a protein. TM-align generates an optimal residue-to-residue alignment based on structural similarity utilizing dynamic programming iterations for two protein structures of uncertain equivalence [38]. TM-score for the five mutated structures shows that they were approximately in the same fold with the normal protein. Figure 4 presents the predicted interatomic interactions calculated for the wild-type protein and the single point mutations. Both wild-type and mutant residues are colored in light green and depicted as sticks, along with domains participating in any interactions surrounding them.

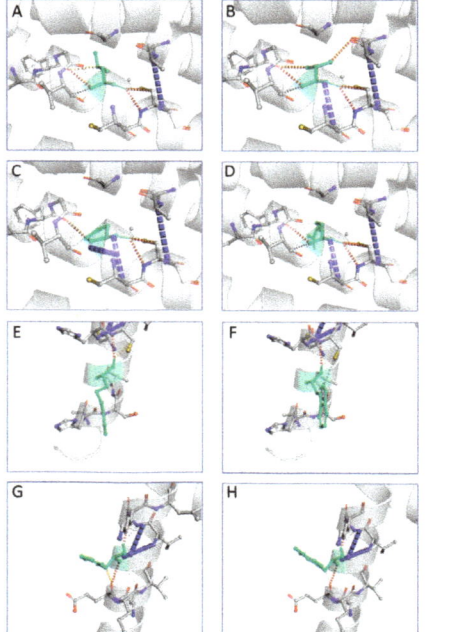

Figure 4. Interatomic interactions for wild-type and mutant PLP1. Both wild-type and mutant residues are colored in light green and depicted as sticks, along with domains participating in any interactions surrounding them. Leucine at position 31 is hydrophobic and highly conserved: (**A**) wild-type residue at position 31; (**B**) L31V (hydrophobic); (**C**) L31P (nonpolar); (**D**) L31R (polar). Arginine at position 137 and histidine at position 140 are polar: (**E**) wild-type residue at position 137; (**F**) R137W (aromatic); (**G**) wild-type residue at position 140; (**H**) H140Y (aromatic). The image is illustrated by DynaMut. A scale of color definition for each type of interaction is provided by software: red depicts hydrogen bonds; slight red depicts water-mediated hydrogen bonds; blue depicts halogen bonds; gold depicts ionic interactions; purple depicts metal complex interactions; light blue depicts aromatic contacts; green depicts hydrophobic contacts; pink depicts carbonyl contacts. The positions of the point mutations are 31, 137 and 140. Abbreviations: L is leucine; P is proline; R is arginine; V is valine; W is tryptophan; H is histidine; Y is tyrosine.

3.8. Validation of the Predicted Structures

The Ramachandran plot was used to examine the conformation of the protein's backbone. It represents an x-y plot of the phi/psi dihedral angles between NC-alpha and Calpha-C bonds. The Ramachandran plot of the wild-type protein in the AlphaFold model revealed 259 residues (94.2%) in the favored regions, 268 (97.5%) in the allowed regions and seven residues in the outlier region (Figure S3). The mutant protein structures obtained by DynaMut demonstrated the same results with wild-type PLP1. On the contrary, I-TASSER structure prediction models display poor Ramachandran plots compared to other algorithms. I-TASSER generates a model by reassembling structural parts from various templates, hence the model occasionally features unfavorable Ramachandran plot regions (Figure S4). The homology models indicated that PLP1 protein models obtained by DynaMut were accurate and they are useful for conducting additional studies and gaining a deeper understanding of the biological activity of the studied protein.

4. Discussion

In this study, the majority of tools indicated that MS-associated PLP1 mutations would have a significant impact on the protein structure, stability and function. Our analysis employed several computational approaches to predict the effects of the PLP1 gene variants, and important results were obtained. Examination of the modified protein structure revealed a destabilizing effect and an increase in flexibility. Loss of protein thermodynamic stability can reduce the ability of its structure to perform normal functions. Furthermore, precise analysis using MutPred2 revealed that these variants may affect protein functionality and structure. We used this machine learning-based approach to integrate data to reason probabilistically about the pathogenicity of amino acid substitutions. The resulted predictions for L31P, L31V and L31R indicated that these mutations may lead to an altered transmembrane protein. The R137W variant may also cause loss of helix, while the H140Y variant may alter the ordered interface of transmembrane protein. The findings of this study provide important insights for future investigations aimed at determining the role of PLP1 in MS.

Missense mutations have a substantial effect on protein functionality. A comprehensive computational examination of the phenotypic characteristics associated with specific variants can reveal the vulnerabilities that interfere with the normal protein activity. This study suggests that mutations in myelin-related genes may play a role in the development of MS. There are two putative PLP1-related MS mechanisms: PLP1 mutations could damage oligodendrocytes [39], generating an inside-out disease process, or they could cause the expression of neoantigens that the immune system could target [14]. Both can occur concurrently, so PLP1 should be investigated further. Previous studies showed that a wide variety of PLP1 genetic alterations have been identified as the underlying causes of PMD and SPG2 [40,41]. Understanding the pathophysiology of the disorders illustrated by a genotype–phenotype correlation requires an understanding of their cellular and metabolic impacts. The consequences of pathological modifications of PLP1 gene were better understood than the physiological functions of the PLP1 protein [37]. After more than 50 years of research, most of the intracellular mechanisms related to PLP1 functionality are still unknown, although the remarkable level of sequence conservation suggests that many mutations could cause severe implications, including MS [14].

In the present study, for most of the known variants, the 3D structures of the proteins are not experimentally known, so there is a clear lack of experimental evaluations of variant effects. Prediction methods can help close the sequence-annotation gap, but with respect to deep annotations of function, in silico methods remain limited. These methods are mainly oriented towards intrinsically disordered proteins and clustered data are based on sequence identity thresholds, retaining a single representative sequence from each group. This approach results in models that resemble having learned a concept instead of a probability distribution. Well-defined theoretical support for this situation is an open problem that will formalize and improve understanding of this long-standing practice in computational biology.

MS is a persistent autoimmune inflammatory disease of the human central nervous system (CNS). It is characterized by loss of motor and sensory function resulting from immune-mediated inflammation, demyelination and sequelae destruction of nerve axons. Along the axon, there are intermittent points that are not surrounded by myelin and are called junctions of Ranvier [42]. MS shows great diversity both at the point of disease onset and at the stage of developmental progression. Four main types of the disease are distinguished: Relapsing–Remitting MS (RRMS) that is characterized by clearly defined relapses of increased disease activity and the worsening of symptoms; Secondary Progressive MS (SPMS), the next step of the RRMS progress for the majority of patients; Primary Progressive MS (PPMS), presenting with symptoms that have been steadily worsening since onset of the disease, without relapses or remissions; and finally Progressive Relapsing MS (PRMS) that is progressive from onset with continuous worsening between relapses [43,44]. Myelin proteins are considered potential targets of the immune system in MS, and activated T-cells recognize specific myelin epitopes at sites of extensive demyelination. According to clinical, pathologic, imaging and electrophysiologic studies, it is not yet understood whether MS is beginning in the periphery, by stimulation of immune cells that thereafter penetrate the CNS and cause damage, or within the CNS through primary myelin or oligodendrocyte injury [45]. This could be the result of mutations in molecules encoding critical components of myelin or oligodendrocytes despite the fact that genome-wide association studies have not found significant links between them and multiple sclerosis. However, it remains possible that mutations in genes encoding these components may be present in a subset of MS patients. In this regard, missense mutations in PLP1 have been identified in patients exhibiting clinical symptoms consistent with a diagnosis of multiple sclerosis [14].

Although the pathogenesis of MS remains unclear, multiple genes, generally of poor penetrance, have been related to MS susceptibility, and their nature suggests autoimmunity causes disease development in most cases [46]. MS is a serious autoimmune disease, unfortunately without a cure; however, over the last three decades, there has been a rapid expansion of therapeutic approaches for the disorder including immunoprotective strategies, shingosine-1-phoshate receptor modulators and cell-based therapies [47]. Emphasis should be placed on early identification of risk factors for early therapeutic interventions. The disease has a different pathogenetic factor in each patient. PLP1 mutations L31V, L31R and R137W could impair PLP trafficking out of the ER and induce the unfolded protein response (UPR). The data imply that PLP1 mutations could have a harmful effect on oligodendrocyte functionality and consequently cause MS [14]. This is confirmed by recent finding in mice carrying the L31R and R137W mutations: they showed neuroinflammation, axonal degeneration, neuronal loss, and brain shrinkage by one year [18]. The same mutations and the loss of function of glial *PLP1* gene indicated a clinical scenario similar to MS in humans. The area of PLP1 gene encoding residue 31 appears to be a hotspot for mutation as L31P has been linked to severe PMD. The L31V mutation shows the least effects on PLP expression, trafficking, or UPR induction is a conservative mutation, as we already stressed [14]. It is not expected to have a significant impact on the hydrophobicity of the first transmembrane region in which it is located, as L and V are hydrophobic amino acids with similar structures and neutral side chains. An L31R mutation in the first transmembrane domain of PLP could affect the overall charge, hydrophobicity, and/or secondary structure of the transmembrane helix, disrupting PLP structure. The L31P mutation would force a stiff bend on the polypeptide and damage the transmembrane helix. R137W occurs in exon 3B, which is deleted in PLP DM20. DM20 is expressed before PLP during ontogenesis and may play a role in the development of new oligodendrocytes [48]. Several L31V-mutated peptides were expected to bind with higher affinity to some of the patient's HLA molecules than the native peptide, producing de novo epitopes and potentially inducing/activating a new group of autoreactive T cells [14,49]. Such responses depend on the presence of proteases that can digest peptides and T cells that can recognize novel epitopes in the patient's T cell repertoire.

5. Conclusions

PLP1 plays an important role in myelin structure and stability, an insulating lipoprotein which helps transmit nerve impulses. Numerous computational tools were utilized in the present in silico analysis, which demonstrated that the amino acid changes L31V, L31R, and R137W of the PLP1 protein are functionally detrimental. The L31V and L31R variants of PLP1 reside in the conserved domain of the protein. To examine the stability of mutant and wild-type PLP1 proteins, we also calculated the changes in their free energies. Our findings provide evidence for the functional role of these three variations, which facilitates the establishment of accurate insights for drug targeting and future clinical application in patients with multiple sclerosis. Alteration of overall cellular activity often arises as a consequence of altered function of one or more individual proteins. Identification of more variants as specific targets may provide a better understanding of conformational dynamics for future studies, while molecular recognition specific to mutated proteins will play an important role in broadening the scope of intracellular mechanisms involved in inflammatory demyelinating diseases.

Key Points

1. The majority of computational tools indicated that MS-associated *PLP1* mutations would have a significant impact on the protein structure, stability and function.
2. Loss of protein thermodynamic stability can reduce the ability of its structure to perform normal functions.
3. The resulted predictions for L31P, L31V and L31R indicated that these mutations may lead to an altered transmembrane protein.
4. The R137W variant may also cause loss of helix, while the H140Y variant may alter the ordered interface of transmembrane protein.

Supplementary Materials: The following supporting information can be downloaded at: https://www.mdpi.com/article/10.3390/brainsci13010042/s1, Table S1: Prediction of pathogenicity of amino acid substitutions of *PLP1* variants; Table S2: Analysis of missense mutations on protein stability; Figure S1: Prediction of evolutionary conserved amino acid residues of PLP1; Figure S2: Protein secondary structure predictions of PLP1; Figure S3 and Figure S4: Ramachandran plots.

Author Contributions: A.A., M.G.K., T.P.E. and P.V. contributed to conceptualization, methodology, data curation, writing—original draft preparation and writing—review and editing. All authors have read and agreed to the published version of the manuscript.

Funding: This research has been co-financed by the European Union and Greek national funds through the Operational Program Competitiveness, Entrepreneurship and Innovation, under the call Regional Excellence (Research Activity in the Ionian University, for the study of protein folding in neurodegenerative diseases) (FOLDIT) MIS 5047144.

Institutional Review Board Statement: Not applicable.

Informed Consent Statement: Not applicable.

Data Availability Statement: Not applicable.

Conflicts of Interest: The authors declare no conflict of interest.

References

1. Salzer, J.L. Schwann cell myelination. *Cold Spring Harb. Perspect. Biol.* **2015**, *7*, a020529. [CrossRef] [PubMed]
2. Poitelon, Y.; Kopec, A.M.; Belin, S. Myelin fat facts: An overview of lipids and fatty acid metabolism. *Cells* **2020**, *9*, 812. [CrossRef] [PubMed]
3. Greer, J.M.; Pender, M.P. Myelin proteolipid protein: An effective autoantigen and target of autoimmunity in multiple sclerosis. *J. Autoimmun.* **2008**, *31*, 281–287. [CrossRef] [PubMed]

4. Greer, J.M.; Trifilieff, E.; Pender, M.P. Correlation between anti-myelin proteolipid protein (PLP) antibodies and disease severity in multiple sclerosis patients with PLP response-permissive HLA types. *Front. Immunol.* **2020**, *11*, 1891. [CrossRef] [PubMed]
5. Mangalam, A.K.; Khare, M.; Krco, C.; Rodriguez, M.; David, C. Identification of T cell epitopes on human proteolipid protein and induction of experimental autoimmune encephalomyelitis in HLA class II-transgenic mice. *Eur. J. Immunol.* **2004**, *34*, 280–290. [CrossRef]
6. Martinsen, V.; Kursula, P. Multiple sclerosis and myelin basic protein: Insights into protein disorder and disease. *Amino Acids* **2021**, *54*, 99–109. [CrossRef]
7. Peschl, P.; Bradl, M.; Höftberger, R.; Berger, T.; Reindl, M. Myelin oligodendrocyte glycoprotein: Deciphering a target in inflammatory demyelinating diseases. *Front. Immunol.* **2017**, *8*, 529. [CrossRef]
8. Quarles, R.H. Myelin-associated glycoprotein (MAG): Past, present and beyond. *J. Neurochem.* **2007**, *100*, 1431–1448. [CrossRef]
9. Rothbard, J.B.; Zhao, X.; Sharpe, O.; Strohman, M.J.; Kurnellas, M.; Mellins, E.D.; Robinson, W.H.; Steinman. L. Chaperone activity of α B-crystallin is responsible for its incorrect assignment as an autoantigen in multiple sclerosis. *J. Immunol.* **2011**, *186*, 4263–4268. [CrossRef]
10. Höftberger, R.; Lassmann, H. Inflammatory demyelinating diseases of the central nervous system. *Handb. Clin. Neurol.* **2018**, *145*, 263–283.
11. Mapunda, J.A.; Tibar, H.; Regragui, W.; Engelhardt, B. How Does the Immune System Enter the Brain? *Front. Immunol.* **2022**, *13*, 805657. [CrossRef] [PubMed]
12. Dhaiban, S.; Al-Ani, M.; Elemam, N.M.; Al-Aawad, M.H.; Al-Rawi, Z.; Maghazachi, A.A. Role of peripheral immune cells in multiple sclerosis and experimental autoimmune encephalomyelitis. *Sci* **2021**, *3*, 12. [CrossRef]
13. Cotsapas, C.; Mitrovic, M. Genome-wide association studies of multiple sclerosis. *Clin. Transl. Immunol.* **2018**, *7*, e1018. [CrossRef] [PubMed]
14. Cloake, N.C.; Yan, J.; Aminian, A.; Pender, M.P.; Greer, J.M. PLP1 mutations in patients with multiple sclerosis: Identification of a new mutation and potential pathogenicity of the mutations. *J. Clin. Med.* **2018**, *7*, 342. [CrossRef]
15. Warshawsky, I.; Rudick, R.A.; Staugaitis, S.M.; Natowicz, M.R. Primary progressive multiple sclerosis as a phenotype of a PLP1 gene mutation. *Ann. Neurol.* **2005**, *58*, 470–473. [CrossRef]
16. Rubegni, A.; Battisti, C.; Tessa, A.; Cerase, A.; Doccini, S.; Santorelli, F.M.; Federico, A. SPG2 mimicking multiple sclerosis in a family identified using next generation sequencing. *J. Neurol. Sci.* **2017**, *375*, 198–202. [CrossRef]
17. Cailloux, F.; Gauthier-Barichard, F.; Mimault, C.; Isabelle, V.; Courtois, V.; Giraud, G.; Dastugue, B.; Boespflug-Tanguy, O.; Clinical European Network on Brain Dysmyelinating Disease. Genotype-phenotype correlation in inherited brain myelination defects due to proteolipid protein gene mutations. *Eur. J. Hum. Genet.* **2000**, *8*, 837–845. [CrossRef]
18. Groh, J.; Friedman, H.C.; Orel, N.; Ip, C.W.; Fischer, S.; Spahn, I.; Schäffner, E.; Hörner, M.; Stadler, D.; Buttmann, M.; et al. Pathogenic inflammation in the CNS of mice carrying human PLP1 mutations. *Hum. Mol. Genet.* **2016**, *25*, 4686–4702.
19. Robert, F.; Pelletier, J. Exploring the impact of single-nucleotide polymorphisms on translation. *Front. Genet.* **2018**, *9*, 507. [CrossRef]
20. Flores, S.C.; Alexiou, A.; Glaros, A. Mining the Protein Data Bank to improve prediction of changes in protein-protein binding. *PLoS ONE* **2021**, *16*, e0257614. [CrossRef]
21. Zerbino, D.R.; Achuthan, P.; Akannietal, W. Ensembl 2018. *Nucleic Acids Res.* **2018**, *46*, D754–D761. [CrossRef] [PubMed]
22. Liu, X.; Jian, X.; Boerwinkle, E. dbNSFP: A lightweight database of human non-synonymous SNPs and their functional predictions. *Hum. Mutat.* **2011**, *32*, 894–899. [CrossRef] [PubMed]
23. Liu, X.; Li, C.; Mou, C.; Dong, Y.; Tu, Y. dbNSFP v4: A comprehensive database of transcript-specific functional predictions and annotations for human nonsynonymous and splice-site SNVs. *Genome Med.* **2020**, *12*, 103. [CrossRef] [PubMed]
24. Pejaver, V.; Urresti, J.; Lugo-Martinez, J.; Pagel, K.A.; Lin, G.N.; Nam, H.; Mort, M.; Cooper, D.N.; Sebat, J.; Iakoucheva, L.M.; et al. Inferring the molecular and phenotypic impact of amino acid variants with MutPred2. *Nat. Commun.* **2020**, *11*, 5918. [CrossRef] [PubMed]
25. Tokuriki, N.; Stricher, F.; Serrano, L.; Tawfik, D.S. How protein stability and new functions trade off. *PLoS Comput. Biol.* **2008**, *4*, e1000002. [CrossRef]
26. Rodrigues, C.H.; Pires, D.E.; Ascher, D.B. DynaMut: Predicting the impact of mutations on protein conformation, flexibility and stability. *Nucleic Acids Res.* **2018**, *46*, W350–W355. [CrossRef]
27. Worth, C.L.; Preissner, R.; Blundell, T.L. SDM—A server for predicting effects of mutations on protein stability and malfunction. *Nucleic Acids Res.* **2011**, *39*, 215–222. [CrossRef]
28. Ashkenazy, H.; Abadi, S.; Martz, E.; Chay, O.; Mayrose, I.; Pupko, T.; Ben-Tal, N. ConSurf 2016: An improved methodology to estimate and visualize evolutionary conservation in macromolecules. *Nucleic Acids Res.* **2016**, *44*, W344–W350. [CrossRef]
29. Buchan, D.W.; Minneci, F.; Nugent, T.C.; Bryson, K.; Jones, D.T. Scalable web services for the PSIPRED protein analysis workbench. *Nucleic Acids Res.* **2013**, *41*, W349–W357. [CrossRef]
30. Arnold, K.; Bordoli, L.; Kopp, J.; Schwede, T. The SWISS-MODEL workspace: A web-based environment for protein structure homology modelling. *Bioinformatics* **2006**, *22*, 195–201. [CrossRef]
31. Kelley, L.A.; Mezulis, S.; Yates, C.M.; Wass, M.N.; Sternberg, M.J. The Phyre2 web portal for protein modeling, prediction and analysis. *Nat. Protoc.* **2015**, *10*, 845–858. [CrossRef] [PubMed]

32. Yang, J.; Yan, R.; Roy, A.; Xu, D.; Poisson, J.; Zhang, Y. The I-TASSER Suite: Protein structure and function prediction. *Nat. Methods* **2015**, *12*, 7–8. [CrossRef] [PubMed]
33. Yang, J.; Zhang, Y. I-TASSER server: New development for protein structure and function predictions. *Nucleic Acids Res.* **2015**, *43*, W174–W181. [CrossRef] [PubMed]
34. Zheng, W.; Zhang, C.; Li, Y.; Pearce, R.; Bell, E.W.; Zhang, Y. Folding non-homology proteins by coupling deep-learning contact maps with I-TASSER assembly simulations. *Cell Rep. Methods* **2021**, *1*, 100014. [CrossRef] [PubMed]
35. Pandit, S.B.; Skolnick, J. Fr-tm-align: A new protein structural alignment method based on fragment alignments and the tm-score. *BMC Bioinform.* **2008**, *9*, 531. [CrossRef]
36. Williams, C.J.; Headd, J.J.; Moriarty, N.W.; Prisant, M.G.; Videau, L.L.; Deis, L.N.; Verma, V.; Keedy, D.A.; Hintze, B.J.; Chen, V.B.; et al. MolProbity: More and better reference data for improved all-atom structure validation. *Protein Sci.* **2018**, *27*, 293–315. [CrossRef]
37. Khalaf, G.; Mattern, C.; Begou, M.; Boespflug-Tanguy, O.; Massaad, C.; Massaad-Massade, L. Mutation of proteolipid protein 1 gene: From severe hypomyelinating leukodystrophy to inherited spastic paraplegia. *Biomedicines* **2022**, *10*, 1709. [CrossRef]
38. Zhang, Y.; Skolnick, J. TM-align: A protein structure alignment algorithm based on the TM-score. *Nucleic Acids Res.* **2005**, *33*, 2302–2309. [CrossRef]
39. Sima, A.A.; Pierson, C.R.; Woltjer, R.L.; Hobson, G.M.; Golden, J.A.; Kupsky, W.J.; Schauer, G.M.; Bird, T.D.; Skoff, R.P.; Garbern, J.Y. Neuronal loss in Pelizaeus–Merzbacher disease differs in various mutations of the proteolipid protein 1. *Acta Neuropathol.* **2009**, *118*, 531–539. [CrossRef]
40. Bonnet-Dupeyron, M.N.; Combes, P.; Santander, P.; Cailloux, F.; Boespflug-Tanguy, O.; Vaurs-Barrière, C. PLP1 splicing abnormalities identified in Pelizaeus-Merzbacher disease and SPG2 fibroblasts are associated with different types of mutations. *Hum. Mutat.* **2008**, *29*, 1028–1036. [CrossRef]
41. Grossi, S.; Regis, S.; Biancheri, R.; Mort, M.; Lualdi, S.; Bertini, E.; Uziel, G.; Boespflug-Tanguy, O.; Simonati, A.; Corsolini, F.; et al. Molecular genetic analysis of the PLP1 gene in 38 families with PLP1-related disorders: Identification and functional characterization of 11 novel PLP1 mutations. *Orphanet J. Rare Dis.* **2011**, *6*, 40. [CrossRef] [PubMed]
42. Lubetzki, C.; Sol-Foulon, N.; Desmazières, A. Nodes of Ranvier during development and repair in the CNS. *Nat. Rev. Neurol.* **2020**, *16*, 426–439. [CrossRef] [PubMed]
43. Klineova, S.; Lublin, F.D. Clinical course of multiple sclerosis. *Cold Spring Harb. Perspect. Med.* **2018**, *8*, a028928. [CrossRef] [PubMed]
44. Cree, B.A.; Arnold, D.L.; Chataway, J.; Chitnis, T.; Fox, R.J.; Ramajo, A.P.; Murphy, N.; Lassmann, H. Secondary progressive multiple sclerosis: New insights. *Neurology* **2021**, *97*, 378–388. [CrossRef] [PubMed]
45. Oudejans, E.; Luchicchi, A.; Strijbis, E.M.; Geurts, J.J.; van Dam, A.M. Is MS affecting the CNS only? Lessons from clinic to myelin pathophysiology. *Neurol. Neuroimmunol. Neuroinflamm.* **2021**, *8*, e914. [CrossRef] [PubMed]
46. Patsopoulos, N.A. Genetics of multiple sclerosis: An overview and new directions. *Cold Spring Harb. Perspect. Med.* **2018**, *8*, a028951. [CrossRef] [PubMed]
47. Yang, J.H.; Rempe, T.; Whitmire, N.; Dunn-Pirio, A.; Graves, J.S. Therapeutic advances in multiple sclerosis. *Front. Neurol.* **2022**, *13*, 824926. [CrossRef]
48. Spörkel, O.; Uschkureit, T.; Büssow, H.; Stoffel, W. Oligodendrocytes expressing exclusively the DM20 isoform of the proteolipid protein gene: Myelination and development. *Glia* **2002**, *37*, 19–30. [CrossRef]
49. Wang, P.; Sidney, J.; Dow, C.; Mothé, B.; Sette, A.; Peters, B. A systematic assessment of MHC class II peptide binding predictions and evaluation of a consensus approach. *PLoS Comput. Biol.* **2008**, *4*, e1000048. [CrossRef]

Disclaimer/Publisher's Note: The statements, opinions and data contained in all publications are solely those of the individual author(s) and contributor(s) and not of MDPI and/or the editor(s). MDPI and/or the editor(s) disclaim responsibility for any injury to people or property resulting from any ideas, methods, instructions or products referred to in the content.

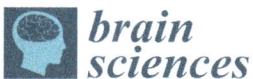

Article

Based on Tau PET Radiomics Analysis for the Classification of Alzheimer's Disease and Mild Cognitive Impairment

Fangyang Jiao [1,†], Min Wang [2,†], Xiaoming Sun [3], Zizhao Ju [1], Jiaying Lu [1], Luyao Wang [2], Jiehui Jiang [2,*] and Chuantao Zuo [1,*]

[1] Department of Nuclear Medicine and PET Center, National Center for Neurological Diseases and National Clinical Research Center for Aging and Medicine, Huashan Hospital, Fudan University, Shanghai 200235, China
[2] Institute of Biomedical Engineering, School of Life Science, Shanghai University, Shanghai 200444, China
[3] School of Communication and Information Engineering, Shanghai University, Shanghai 200444, China
* Correspondence: jiangjiehui@shu.edu.cn (J.J.); zuochuantao@fudan.edu.cn (C.Z.)
† These authors contributed equally to this work.

Abstract: Alzheimer's Disease (AD) and Mild Cognitive Impairment (MCI) are closely associated with Tau proteins accumulation. In this study, we aimed to implement radiomics analysis to discover high-order features from pathological biomarker and improve the classification accuracy based on Tau PET images. Two cross-racial independent cohorts from the ADNI database (121 AD patients, 197 MCI patients and 211 normal control (NC) subjects) and Huashan hospital (44 AD patients, 33 MCI patients and 36 NC subjects) were enrolled. The radiomics features of Tau PET imaging of AD related brain regions were computed for classification using a support vector machine (SVM) model. The radiomics model was trained and validated in the ADNI cohort and tested in the Huashan hospital cohort. The standard uptake value ratio (SUVR) and clinical scores model were also performed to compared with radiomics analysis. Additionally, we explored the possibility of using Tau PET radiomics features as a good biomarker to make binary identification of Tau-negative MCI versus Tau-positive MCI or apolipoprotein E (ApoE) ε4 carrier versus ApoE ε4 non-carrier. We found that the radiomics model demonstrated best classification performance in differentiating AD/MCI patients and NC in comparison to SUVR and clinical scores models, with an accuracy of 84.8 ± 4.5%, 73.1 ± 3.6% in the ANDI cohort. Moreover, the radiomics model also demonstrated greater performance in diagnosing AD than other methods in the Huashan hospital cohort, with an accuracy of 81.9 ± 6.1%. In addition, the radiomics model also showed the satisfactory classification performance in the MCI-tau subgroup experiment (72.3 ± 3.5%, 71.9 ± 3.6% and 63.7 ± 5.9%) and in the MCI-ApoE subgroup experiment (73.5 ± 4.3%, 70.1 ± 3.9% and 62.5 ± 5.4%). In conclusion, our study showed that based on Tau PET radiomics analysis has the potential to guide and facilitate clinical diagnosis, further providing evidence for identifying the risk factors in MCI patients.

Keywords: Tau PET; radiomics; Alzheimer's Disease; Mild Cognitive Impairment

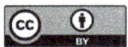

1. Introduction

Alzheimer's Disease (AD) is a common neurodegenerative disease marked by chronic primary progressive memory decline and cognitive impairment, which is one of the most serious diseases threatening the elderly [1]. At present, the early identification and accurate diagnosis for prodromal AD are crucial for clinical decision-making and future development of treatments. Mild Cognitive Impairment (MCI), as a prodromal stage of AD, remains the most common underlying AD pathology or mixed pathology [2]. In line with the latest A-T-N framework, pathologic Tau is closely associated with neurodegeneration and necessary for AD-related downstream events [3–5]. Quantifiable tau loads and its corresponding increase may be a relevant target engagement marker for clinical disease-modifying interventions in anti-Tau agents.

Positron emission tomography (PET) offers the opportunity for non-invasively detecting regional distribution of Tau pathology at early stages of neurodegenerative disorders. First-generation Tau PET ligands have been developed as a highly credible biomarker of 3R/4R Tau deposits [6]. For instance, ^{18}F-flortaucipir (known as ^{18}F-AV-1451) PET pattern in AD/MCI specifically targets the clinically affected brain regions (e.g., medial temporal and lateral temporoparietal regions) and shows a strong regional association with domain-specific neuropsychological tests [7]. New Tau PET ligands (e.g., ^{18}F-MK-6240, ^{18}F-PI-2620 and ^{18}F-Florzolotau (also known as ^{18}F-APN-1607 and ^{18}F-PM-PBB3) overcome the off-target binding of the first-generation products and provide fresh insight on the time course of Tau accumulation related to other biomarkers and clinical manifestation [8,9]. The application of qualitative and quantitative measure of Tau PET imaging, on the other hand, is in its early stages. The existing PET biomarker and corresponding "defined cutoffs" may not always reflect the presence or absence of pathology. One Tau-negative study estimate that 27.5% of MCI or dementia due to AD in those >75 years of age might be Tau-PET negative [10]. At this time, it is unknown how much pathologic Tau can be present in the brain below the in vivo Tau PET detectable threshold. As the most popular qualitative and quantitative analysis for PET imaging, visual reading and standard uptake value ratio (SUVR) may necessitate the sacrifice for complete information in relation to underlying regional Tau protein deposition. We anticipate that minimal neurofibrillary changes that are detectable by neuropathology examination can also be identified by Tau PET. Moreover, some studies have confirmed that brain Tau PET signal changes with age in cognitively unimpaired individuals and AD patients [11–13]. Tau pathology accumulates early in aging and relentlessly progresses in the course of AD. These limitations bring challenges to the clinical utilization of Tau PET imaging.

Radiomics analysis can be applied to explore previously unrecognized signs and patterns of disease evolution and progression by transforming image data into high-throughput features that are difficult to detect by the visual system or intensity-based metrics [14]. Until now, it has been applied to a variety of neuropsychiatric diseases including AD/MCI. Previous studies including MRI, ^{18}F- fluoro-2-deoxyglucose (^{18}F-FDG) PET and Amyloid β-protein (Aβ) PET have shown that radiomics features and classification models have potential as biomarkers for the diagnosis of AD and MCI [15–18]. These provide important imaging information for the heterogeneity distribution of microstructure, metabolism and pathological Aβ in AD or MCI. However, there is no similar research to deeply explore Tau neuropathological profile. It is also debatable whether radiomics analysis can be employed in Tau-negative PET images. The apolipoprotein E (ApoE) ε4 gene has been identified as a significant genetic risk factor for AD/MCI [19]. Previous results found associations between the gene expression and the deposition of Tau for AD [19]. The relationships between Tau PET radiomics features and genetic expression are not well understood.

Considering the important role of Tau deposits in clinical symptoms and pathological revelations [20] and the ability of radiomics in high-throughput mining of image features, we hypothesizes that based on Tau PET radiomics analysis may also be dynamic in the classification of AD and MCI patients. Furthermore, we anticipate that this method will be used as neuroimaging biomarkers to differentiate patients with risk factors. Hence, the first objective of this study is to propose and validate Tau-based radiomics features model for diagnosing AD/MCI patients by different cohorts (Alzheimer Disease Neuroimaging Initiative (ADNI)-Huashan hospital) and different Tau PET tracers (^{18}F-AV1451-^{18}F-Florzolotau). Additionally, we explored the possibility of using radiomics features as a good biomarker to make binary identification of Tau-negative MCI versus Tau-positive MCI or ApoE ε4 carrier versus ApoE ε4 non-carrier, which is of significant importance, but limited for clinical tests.

2. Materials and Methods

Figure 1 shows the overall workflow of Tau PET radiomics analysis, namely, (A) collection of images and division of subgroups, (B) image preprocessing, (C) identification regions of interest (ROIs), (D) feature extraction and selection and (E) SVM classification.

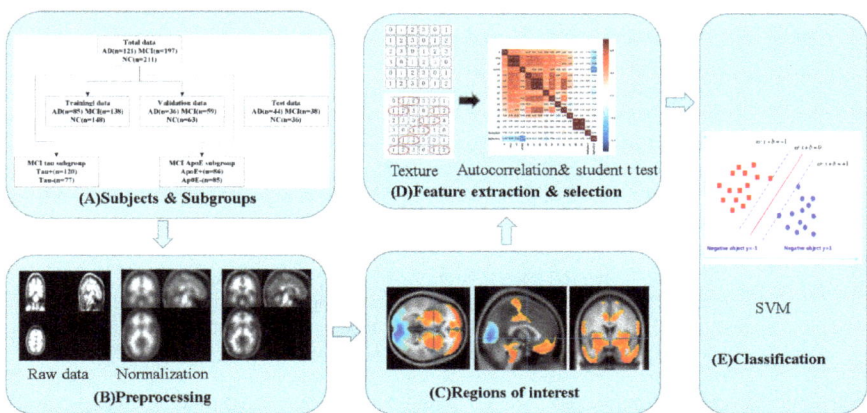

Figure 1. The main workflow for Tau PET radiomics analysis comprised five sections: subjects, subgroups, preprocessing, regions of interest and classification. SVM: support vector machine.

2.1. Subjects

All subjects were collected from two different cohorts: ADNI database and Huashan hospital, Fudan university. (1) For ADNI cohort, 121 AD patients, 197 MCI patients and 211 normal control (NC) subjects were enrolled from ADNI-1, ADNI-2, ADNI-3 and ANDI GO. Detailed subject inclusion information for ADNI cohort can be found at http://adni.loni.usc.edu (accessed on 3 May 2022). (2) For Huashan hospital cohort, 44 AD patients, 33 MCI patients and 36 NC subjects were enrolled. AD or MCI patients from Huashan hospital were clinically evaluated and judged by senior neurologists of cognitive disorders based on the current diagnostic guidelines [21,22]. NC subjects had no history for neurologic and psychiatric disorders, and no abnormal neurological examination.

For ADNI and Huashan hospital cohort, age, gender, years of education and Mini-Mental State Examination (MMSE) score were recorded. Imaging data, including ^{18}F-flortaucipir (ADNI only) PET, ^{18}F-florzolotau PET (Huashan hospital only) and T1-weighted structural MRI were collected. Table 1 shows the basic characteristics of all the subjects.

Table 1. Demographic, clinical characteristics for ANDI cohort and Huashan hospital subjects.

	Age (Years)	Sex (Male/Female)	Education (Years)	MMSE
ANDI cohort				
AD (n = 121)	72.1 ± 7.5 *	55/66 *	15.5 ± 2.6 *	24.0 ± 3.3 *
MCI (n = 197)	71.1 ± 7.4 †	108/89 †	16.4 ± 2.5 †	27.9 ± 1.9 †‡
NC (n = 211)	71.2 ± 6.4	79/132	16.7 ± 2.3	29.1 ± 1.2
Huashan hospital				
AD (n = 44)	58.2 ± 9.6	17/27	9.8 ± 4.2 *	16.6 ± 6.9 *
MCI (n = 33)	69.4 ± 8.4 †‡	10/23	10.4 ± 3.2 †	25.6 ± 1.8 †‡
NC (n = 36)	58.5 ± 8.2	18/20	10.1 ± 2.1	27.2 ± 2.5

Data are given as numbers or mean ± standard deviation (SD) values. * $p < 0.05$ AD vs. NC. † $p < 0.05$ MCI vs. NC. ‡ $p < 0.05$ AD vs. MCI. MMSE: Mini-Mental State Examination.

The ADNI cohort was approved by the institutional review board at each site and all the participants provided their written consent. The institutional review board of Huashan Hospital (HIRB) granted ethics approval for Huashan hospital cohort (No. 2018-363). All patients from Huashan hospital provided written informed consent.

2.2. Radiomics Model

Image Acquisition and preprocessing

Subjects in ADNI and Huashan cohort were scanned by structural T1 MRI and Tau PET. Detailed information about the ANDI acquisition protocol is described on the website (http://adni.loni.usc.edu/ accessed on 3 May 2022). Participants from Huashan hospital underwent a 3.0-T anatomical MRI (Discovery MR750; GE Medical Systems, Milwaukee, WI, USA) with FOV = 25.6 cm, matrix = $256 \times 256 \times 152$, slice thickness = 1 mm, repetition time (TR) = 8.2 ms, echo time (TE) = 3.2 ms, flip angle= $12°$. 18F-Florzolotau PET were acquired on a Siemens mCT Flow PET/CT scanner (Siemens, Erlangen, Germany) in three-dimensional (3D) mode over a 20 min acquisition time (90–110 min) and reconstructed by the ordered subset expectation maximization (OSEM) method. The detailed acquisition protocol for Huanshan hospital has been reported in our previous study [23].

All PET images preprocessing were performed in MATLAB R2018a (MathWorks, Natick, MA, USA) using the Statistical Parametric Mapping toolbox (version 12; http://www.fil.ion.ucl.ac.uk/spm/software/spm12/ accessed on 9 May 2022). Frist, PET images were co-registered with corresponding T1-weighted MRI images. Second, co-registered PET images were normalized to the Montreal Neurological Institute (MNI) space using the forward the spatial transformation matrix. Third, normalized PET images were subsequently smoothed with a Gaussian kernel with a full width at half maximum of 8 mm to blur image edges and improve the signal-to-noise ratio.

Definition of ROIs

For Tau PET, we concentrated on brain areas associated with AD-related Tau protein deposition, and defined these ROIs to obtain more detailed radiomics features. Namely, a group comparison using a two-sample t test between AD and NC from ANDI training datasets (including 85 AD patients and 148 NC subjects) were performed to define the ROIs with significant differences (FDR corrected, $p < 0.01$ and cluster size > 500). These ROIs were mapped to Automated Anatomical Labeling (AAL) for localization by xjView9.6 (http://www.alivelearn.net/xjview accessed on 23 May 2022). As MCI remains the most common underlying AD pathology or mixed pathology, we assume that these ROIs overlap MCI-related brain areas and can also be used to extract MCI radiomics features. Furthermore, the AD related regions were considered as ROIs to maintain consistency of radiomics analysis in subsequent studies.

Radiomics Feature Extraction and Selection

For each subject, radiomics features from each AD related ROIs were computed by a MATLAB toolkit for radiomics analysis (https://github.com/mvallieres/radiomics/ accessed on 6 June 2022). First, the Lloyd-Max quantization algorithm was applied to normalize the preprocessed PET images for isotropic resampling. Second, radiomics features were calculated from quantized PET images. Finally, 3 features from first-order histogram, 9 features from the Gray-Level Co-occurrence Matrix (GLCM), 13 features from the Gray-Level Run-Length Matrix (GLRLM), 13 features from the Gray-Level Size Zone Matrix (GLSZM) and 5 features from the Neighborhood Gray-Tone Difference Matrix (NGTDM) were extracted. Global features were extracted from the intensity histogram of the ROIs, whereas GLCM, GLRLM, GLSZM and NGTDM textures are matrix-based features. The detailed mathematical definition of the radiomics matrices were previously reported [18].

After feature extraction, two steps were performed for features selection: (1) Correlation analysis was first performed to reduce the dimensionality. If the correlation coefficient of two feature columns exceeded 0.1, we removed one of them randomly. (2) Second, a two-sample student's t test between AD and NC from ANDI training datasets (including

85 AD patients and 148 NC subjects) were used to further select the features with significant differences ($p < 0.005$).

Classification

The subjects from ADNI data were randomly assigned to training and validation datasets at proportions of 0.7 and 0.3, respectively. The SVM was applied to construct the classification models of the AD-NC and MCI-NC groups based on the selected features with five-fold cross-validation 100 times in training datasets and the validation dataset was used to verify the robustness of our radiomics model. Then, the data from Huashan hospital were used as independent external test sets to validate the reliability and robustness of the corresponding models. In addition, age and sex had been treated as the covariates for SVM classification. Receiver operating characteristic (ROC) curves and the corresponding areas under the curve (AUC) were used to evaluate the diagnostic capabilities of the radiomics features.

2.3. Comparative Models

To verify the superiority of radiomics model, two comparative models were performed as the followed: (1) SUVR model: the SUVR value of each ROI was calculated by a reference region (cerebellum) and used as the input of the classifier. (2) Clinical scores model: MMSE scores, as the inputs, were construct the clinical prediction model. The SVM with a linear kernel function was also used as the classifier in the comparative experiment.

2.4. Radiomics Model in MCI Subgroups

To explore the performance of radiomics model on the identification of Tau-negative MCI vs. Tau-positive MCI or MCI ApoE ε4 carrier vs. ApoE ε4 non-carrier, MCI patients were further divided into subgroups. (1) For Tau-negative MCI vs. Tau-positive MCI(MCI-tau (+)/MCI-tau(-)), MCI Tau PET images were visually interpreted by two experienced neuroimaging specialist who were blinded to clinical information and made positive or negative decisions based global cortical binding. The final binary decision was based on the consensus of two independent assessors. (2) For ApoE ε4 carrier vs. ApoE ε4 non-carrier (MCI-ApoE(+)/MCI-ApoE(-)), ApoE gene expression was recorded only in 171 MCI patients from ANDI cohort. The ApoE status was determined by the ApoE ε4 gene expression or not. Radiomics model was treated with the same method as above.

2.5. Statistical Analysis

Statistical analyses were performed using SPSS software 26.0 (IBM Corporation, Armonk, NY, USA). For categorical and continuous variables, the demographic information was collected as numbers or means ± SD. The chi-squared tests for categorical variables (sex) and one-way ANOVA test between AD, MCI and NC groups was performed. Values were considered significant for $p < 0.05$.

3. Results

3.1. Demographic and Clinical Characteristics

The demographic and clinical characteristics of the ANDI cohort and Huashan hospital subjects are presented in Table 1. (1) For the ANDI cohort, there was a significant difference in age, sex, years of education and MMSE between AD and NC or MCI and NC group ($p < 0.05$) and the AD group is different from MCI group in MMSE scores ($p < 0.05$). There is no difference in age, sex or years of education between AD and MCI group. (2) For Huashan hospital cohort, a difference in age, years of education and MMSE between MCI and NC group ($p < 0.05$) and a difference in years of education and MMSE between AD and NC group ($p < 0.05$) and there was a difference in age and MMSE between AD and MCI group ($p < 0.05$). There is no age difference between AD and MCI group. No difference was found in sex among the AD, MCI and NC group.

3.2. The Defined ROIs and Selected Features

In final, 60 ROIs based on AAL atlas were obtained from the above method (Table S1). The result showed that majority of the ROIs were found in the frontal, temporal and occipital lobe (Figure 2).

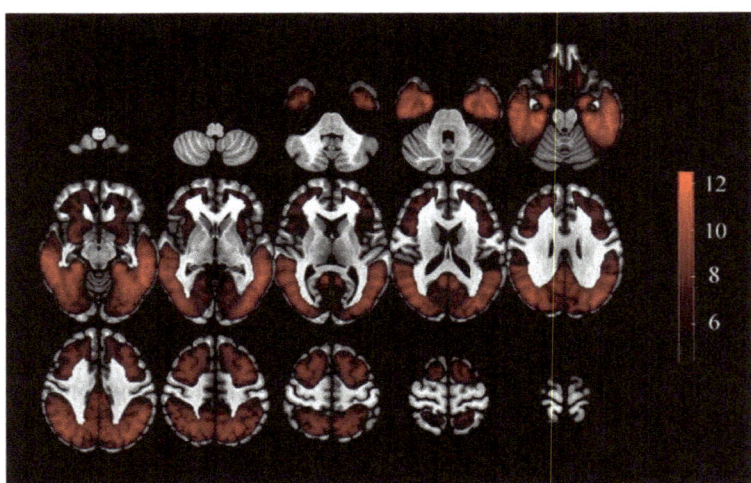

Figure 2. The ROIs related brain regions defined by a two-sample t test between AD and NC from ANDI training datasets. Color bars represent t value. ROIs: Regions of interest.

The total amount of features extracted from ROIs was 2580 ((3 + 40) × 60 = 2580). After the features selection, 31 features mainly from GLSZM and NGTDM were left in the frontal, temporal and occipital lobe. The details of these features provided in Table S2.

3.3. Tau PET Radiomics Model for the Diagnosis AD/MCI

For the identification of AD from NC, we obtained an accuracy of 84.8 ± 4.5% with the ADNI validation dataset by radiomics model and an accuracy of 81.9 ± 6.1% with the Huashan hospital as the independent external test data. The performances of the SUVR and Clinical scores model were poorer than radiomics model with accuracies of 80.3 ± 1.4% and 70.5 ± 5.2%, respectively, in the ADNI validation dataset and 75.1 ± 3.5% and 66.4 ± 10.2%, respectively, in the Huashan hospital cohort (Table 2).

Table 2. The classification results for AD vs. NC subjects.

Model	Accuracy (%)	Sensibility (%)	Specificity (%)
Radiomics			
Validation	84.8 ± 4.5	76.1 ± 5.1	88.7 ± 2.9
Test	81.9 ± 6.1	83.8 ± 4.9	78.6 ± 7.3
SUVR			
Validation	80.3 ± 1.4	61.5 ± 3.5	87.0 ± 5.0
Test	75.1 ± 3.5	60.8 ± 7.8	79.1 ± 1.5
Clinical scores			
Validation	70.5 ± 5.2	58.2 ± 13.9	79.9 ± 12.0
Test	66.4 ± 10.2	53.3 ± 6.5	70.2 ± 11.7

For the identification of MCI from NC, we obtained an accuracy of 73.1 ± 3.6% with the ADNI validation dataset. The performances of the SUVR and Clinical scores model were poorer than radiomics model with accuracies of 70.8 ± 2.7% and 65.1 ± 5.2%, respectively, in ADNI validation dataset. The accuracy with the Huashan hospital as the independent external test data was 63.5 ± 8.7%. The performances of Clinical scores model (accuracy: 63.1 ± 11.0%) were very similar to radiomics model in the Huashan hospital. However, the performances of the SUVR model (accuracy: 68.7 ± 5.5%) were not poorer than radiomics model (Table 3).

Table 3. The classification results for MCI vs. NC subjects.

Model	Accuracy (%)	Sensibility (%)	Specificity (%)
Radiomics			
Validation	73.1 ± 3.6	71.3 ± 6.1	75.0 ± 5.5
Test	63.5 ± 8.7	65.7 ± 8.8	60.6 ± 5.8
SUVR			
Validation	70.8 ± 2.7	58.5 ± 14.8	88.4 ± 9.8
Test	68.7 ± 5.5	53.8 ± 14.4	86.7 ± 8.7
Clinical scores			
Validation	65.1 ± 5.2	42.5 ± 13.9	87.5 ± 12.0
Test	63.1 ± 11.0	49.8 ± 9.6	80.5 ± 21.5

Compared to SUVR or Clinical scores model, the median AUC of the radiomics model reached 0.906/0.850 and achieved the best performance for diagnosis AD/MCI from NC (Figure 3).

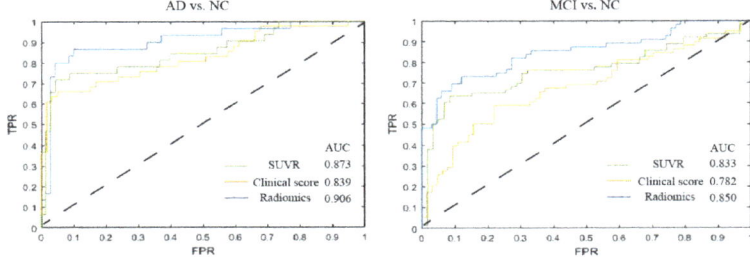

Figure 3. Receiver operating characteristic (ROC) curves in classification of AD vs. NC [AUC: SUVR 0.873 (0.847–0.913), Clinical score 0.839 (0.796–0.962), Radiomics 0.906 (0.850–0.933)] and MCI vs. NC [AUC: SUVR 0.833 (0.797–0.859), Clinical score 0.782 (0.729–0.851), Radiomics 0.850 (0.802–0.911)]. Data are given as median (interquartile range). TPR: True Positive Rate; FPR: False Positive Rate; AUC: Areas under the curve.

3.4. Tau PET Radiomics Model for the Diagnosis MCI Subgroups

With the MCI-tau(+) vs. NC classification, we obtained an accuracy of 93.5 ± 2.7% and 72.3 ± 3.5% for the ADNI training data and validation data, respectively. With the MCI-tau(-) vs. NC classification, the accuracy in the training data and validation data was 91.7 ± 0.9% and 71.9 ± 3.6%, respectively. The performance of the MCI-tau(+) vs. MCI-tau(-) classification was also excellent with the accuracies of 83.4 ± 5.2% and 63.7 ± 5.9% in ADNI training data and validation data, respectively (Table 4.). The AUC for MCI-tau(+) vs. NC, MCI-tau(-) vs. NC and MCI-tau(+) and MCI-tau(-) were 0.918 (0.829–0.955), 0.820 (0.752–0.907) and 0.711 (0.668–0.805), respectively (Figure 4).

For the identification of MCI-ApoE(+) from NC, we obtained an accuracy of 92.7 ± 1.1% and 73.5 ± 4.3% with the ADNI training data and validation data, respectively. For the identification of MCI-ApoE(-) from NC, we obtained an accuracy of 92.5 ± 2.9% and 70.1 ± 3.9% with the ADNI training data and validation data, respectively. In addition, we obtained an accuracy of 87.1 ± 8.9% and 62.5 ± 5.4% for the classification of MCI-ApoE(+) vs. MCI-ApoE(-) (Table 5). The AUC for MCI-ApoE(+) vs. NC, MCI-ApoE(-) vs.

NC and MCI-ApoE(+) and MCI-ApoE(-) were 0.910 (0.861–0.937), 0.826 (0.788–0.853) and 0.701 (0.632–0.747), respectively (Figure 4).

Table 4. The classification results for MCI-tau subgroups.

	Accuracy (%)	Sensibility (%)	Specificity (%)
MCI-tau(+) vs. NC			
Train	93.5 ± 2.7	92.0 ± 2.2	94.1 ± 3.6
Validation	72.3 ± 3.5	70.4 ± 5.9	74.0 ± 5.8
MCI-tau(-) vs. NC			
Train	91.7 ± 0.9	91.0 ± 1.2	92.0 ± 3.4
Validation	71.9 ± 3.6	70.1 ± 6.0	73.5 ± 5.1
MCI-tau(+) vs. MCI-tau(+)			
Train	83.4 ± 5.2	88.5 ± 7.3	80.1 ± 4.5
Validation	63.7 ± 5.9	69.4 ± 6.6	53.2 ± 8.0

Table 5. The classification results for MCI-ApoE subgroups.

	Accuracy (%)	Sensibility (%)	Specificity (%)
MCI-ApoE(+) vs. NC			
Train	92.7 ± 1.1	92.7 ± 2.1	93.8 ± 1.8
Validation	73.5 ± 4.3	68.0 ± 3.8	76.6 ± 4.6
MCI-ApoE(-) vs. NC			
Train	92.5 ± 2.9	91.0 ± 3.3	92.9 ± 2.0
Validation	70.1 ± 3.9	68.0 ± 3.0	72.8 ± 5.1
MCI-ApoE(+) vs. MCI-ApoE(-)			
Train	87.1 ± 8.9	90.3 ± 10.5	83.6 ± 5.7
Validation	62.5 ± 5.4	71.6 ± 7.2	51.6 ± 11.0

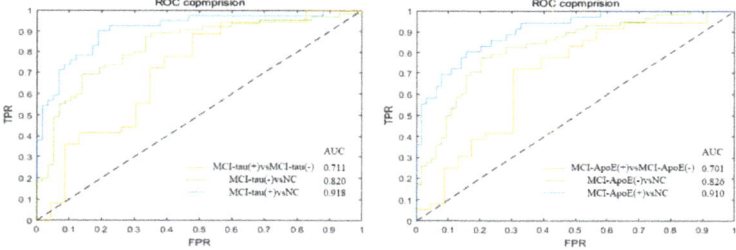

Figure 4. Receiver operating characteristic (ROC) curves in classification of MCI-tau subgroups and MCI-ApoE subgroups. [MCI-tau(+)-MCI-tau(-) AUC: 0.711 (0.668–0.805), MCI-tau(-)-NC AUC: 0.820 (0.752–0.907), MCI-tau(+)-NC AUC: 0.918 (0.829–0.955)]; [MCI-ApoE(+)-MCI-ApoE(-) AUC: 0.701 (0.632–0.747), MCI-ApoE(-)-NC AUC: 0.826 (0.788–0.853) and MCI-ApoE(+)-NC AUC: 0.910 (0.861–0.937)]. Data are given as median (interquartile range). TPR: True Positive Rate; FPR: False Positive Rate; AUC: Areas under the curve.

4. Discussion

So far, few studies had investigated the use of artificial intelligence on Tau PET images for the assessment of neurodegenerative diseases. In this paper, we proposed Tau PET-based radiomics analysis as a novel biomarker to apply to AD/MCI. Meanwhile, we selected two cross-racial independent cohorts with different PET scanners, two imaging tracers, to prove the stability and generalization of the method. We find that this radiomics model has the potential of improving the diagnostic accuracy for AD/MCI, even contributing to the identification of MCI with negative or positive Tau PET. Moreover, we evaluated this model could predict the ApoE4 carrier results of MCI patients, which is an important risk factor predicting progression to dementia.

Radiomics seeks to extract high-throughput quantitative information from medical images, especially those that are difficult for the human eyes to recognize or quantify [14]. Prior studies offered solid evidence that AD/MCI patients had Tau deposition in the frontal, temporal, parietal and occipital lobes [24,25]. In our study, AD-related ROIs were characterized by SPM analysis in frontal, temporal and occipital lobe, which is consistent with those reported in the above literature. Eventually, 31 radiomics features, mainly from GLSZM and NGTDM, in the temporal, parietal, occipital lobes and cingulate gyrus were left. The GLSZM-derived features assess the variability of gray-level intensity values and the distribution of large area size zones in the image [26]. The NGTDM-derived features mainly reflect the difference between a gray value and the average gray value of its neighbors [26]. These radiomics features were usually difficult to detect by manual inspection, but computer-aided technology scan effectively identified them. Significant differences on the above features showed the highest inter-patient variability within the distributions of voxel values. Additionally, it provided multidimensional evidence that Tau deposit occurred in specific brain regions.

Currently, more evidence highlighted the possibility that radiomics can be employed as imaging biomarkers for AD and MCI [27,28]. T1-weighted Magnetic Resonance Imaging (MRI) radiomics methods were first used to distinguish AD/MCI from NC. Other MRI sequences, including Voxel-Based Morphometry (VBM), Susceptibility-Weighted Imaging (SWI) and Diffusion Tensor Imaging (DTI), were used in detecting the brain structural and functional changes of AD and MCI [27]. For example, Feng et al., performed the logistic analysis with a classification accuracy of 0.9 for AD vs. NC, an accuracy of 0.81 for AD vs. MCI and an accuracy of 0.75 for MCI vs. NC [29]. For FDG PET, radiomics features provided the best performance with classification accuracy of 0.77 vary to 0.94 on MCI/NC and AD/NC [18,30]. As the common $A\beta$ neurobiological biomarkers, the high-order features of $A\beta$ PET also achieved an accuracy of 0.87 for AD vs. NC classification [31]. Compared with above studies, our Tau PET radiomics model achieved similar to classification accuracy. Additionally, the classification accuracy remained slightly lower in independent external test dataset from the Huashan hospital cohort. Notably, the Tau PET tracer in Huashan hospital cohort is different from ANDI cohort. Thus, we can conclude that the high accuracy achieved was a consequence of the robustness of the radiomics classification model. According to our results of the comparative experiment, the performance of this model outperformed SUVR or Clinical scores model. For Tau PET, SUVR typically defined as the ratio of average activity in brain ROI relative to reference (usually in cerebellum). However, the reference in cerebellum has some disadvantages including small size, low signal detection sensitivity and the partial volume effect (PVE) [32]. For MMSE scores, it has shown not to be adequate in detecting MCI and clinical signs of dementia due to the ceiling or the floor effect and higher subjectivity [33]. Hence, the incomplete characteristics of the SUVR, limitation of the neuropsychological scales may lead to the comparative results [34].

Variations in the types, amounts and distribution of concomitant AD or non-AD pathologies may account for the Tau 'positivity' or 'negativity' of MCI [35]. Previous studies showed that these Tau negativity individuals were less likely to have AD-related clinical features and that the majority did not develop dementia over at least 5 years of follow-up [36]. Early in vivo diagnosis of MCI with Tau positivity, which may evolve into AD, is critical for accurate patient management. In our study, the radiomics models exhibited satisfactory performance in automated detection of MCI with Tau-negative or Tau-positive cases with mean accuracy of 72.3% or 71.9% from NC. This method could be helpful to identify and eventually treat patients as early as possible in the disease process. It also could be applied to overcome obvious shortcomings of traditional assessment, such as manual operations of image intensity and inter-reader variability of visual interpretation.

The APOE $\varepsilon 4$ genotype expression is related to higher risk of AD/MCI [37]. The associations between the genetic phenotypes and AD-associated Tau deposition had been proven and light the genetic basis for Tau deposition [38]. Considering the toxicity, identification of APOE ε4 carriers and blocking its action may delay or stop the development of AD [39]. As expected, our study showed that radiomics features was also affected by the ApoE ε4 genotype. This radiomics model showed the high accuracy for the identification of APOE ε4 carrier or non-carrier from NC. It is meaningful that Tau radiomics features had been confirmed to have genetic significance and were helpful for identifying MCI with risk genetic factor.

For this study, we draw attention to some limitations. First, the diagnosis of AD/MCI was not confirmed by the autopsy. AD is a significant heterogeneous disease with various forms clinical presentation, which is now referred to as the Alzheimer spectrum [40]. We strictly adopted the standardized clinical diagnostic criteria to classify patients into AD and MCI. Second, we divided MCI subjects into MCI-tau(+) and MCI-tau(-) group by visual interpretation. Considering subjectivity of the naked eye, a reliable strategy for tau PET analysis is desired to be developed in the future. Third, we did not use the scale for related exclusion study. Whether the bias of the scale has an impact on the results needs further discussion. Fourth, we only employed single independent external cohorts with relatively small the number of subjects. A larger cohort and a multicenter study is required for stronger verification in future research. Finally, the study is its retrospective nature. Ongoing longitudinal observational studies in the model will be explored to validate these results.

5. Conclusions

In conclusion, we explored radiomics model for the classification of AD/MCI based on Tau deposition. Our results demonstrated that this model could acquire high-level evidence for clinical practice and accurately and stably identify AD/MCI from NC. In addition, we also find that these radiomics features can identify the risk factors in MCI patients, i.e., deposition of Tau and APOE ε4 gene expression. These findings show that Tau PET radionics can serve as new neuroimaging biomarker for clinical aided classification, further providing evidence that advanced machine learning methods may contribute to clarify the neuropathological mechanism for AD from a new perspective.

Supplementary Materials: The following supporting information can be downloaded at: https://www.mdpi.com/article/10.3390/brainsci13020367/s1, Table S1: 60 ROIs with significant differences between AD and NC from ANDI training datasets on AAL atlas; Table S2: Selected features from ADNI cohorts.

Author Contributions: Conceptualization, J.J. and C.Z.; methodology, M.W. and X.S.; formal analysis, M.W., X.S. and F.J.; data curation, F.J.; writing—original draft preparation, F.J.; writing—review and editing, M.W., X.S., Z.J., J.L., L.W., J.J. and C.Z.; supervision, J.J. and C.Z.; funding acquisition, M.W., L.W. and C.Z. All authors have read and agreed to the published version of the manuscript.

Funding: This research was funded by National Natural Science Foundation of China (No. 82021002, 81971641, 81671239 and 62206165); Research project of Shanghai Health Commission (No. 2020YJZX0111); Clinical Research Plan of SHDC (No. SHDC2020CR1038B); Science and Technology Innovation 2030 Major Projects (No. 2022ZD0211600); Shanghai Science and Technology Development Funds (No. Sailing Program 22YF1413900); China postdoctoral Science Foundation (No. 2022M722034).

Institutional Review Board Statement: The study was conducted in accordance with the Declaration of Helsinki and approved by the Institutional Review Board of Huashan Hospital (HIRB) (No. 2018-363).

Informed Consent Statement: Informed consent was obtained from all subjects involved in the study.

Data Availability Statement: The datasets generated during and/or analyzed during the current study are available from the corresponding author on reasonable request.

Acknowledgments: We are grateful to APRINOIA Therapeutics for the provision of the 18F-Florzolotau precursor.

Conflicts of Interest: The authors declare no conflict of interest. The funders had no role in the design of the study; in the collection, analyses, or interpretation of data; in the writing of the manuscript; or in the decision to publish the results.

Abbreviations

AD	Alzheimer's Disease
MCI	Mild Cognitive Impairment
NC	Normal control
SVM	Support vector machine
SUVR	Standard uptake value ratio
PET	Positron emission tomography
^{18}F-FDG	^{18}F- fluoro-2-deoxyglucose
ApoE	apolipoprotein E
Aβ	Amyloid β-protein
ROIs	Regions of interest
ADNI	Alzheimer Disease Neuroimaging Initiative
MMSE	Mini-Mental State Examination
GLCM	Gray-Level Co-occurrence Matrix
GLRLM	Gray-Level Run-Length Matrix
GLSZM	Gray-Level Size Zone Matrix
NGTDM	Neighborhood Gray-Tone Difference Matrix
ROC	Receiver operating characteristic
AUC	Areas under the curve

References

1. Jack, C.R.; Bennett, D.A.; Blennow, K.; Carrillo, M.C.; Dunn, B.; Haeberlein, S.B.; Holtzman, D.M.; Jagust, W.; Jessen, F.; Karlawish, J.; et al. NIA-AA Research Framework: Toward a biological definition of Alzheimer's disease. *Alzheimer's Dement.* **2018**, *14*, 535–562. [CrossRef] [PubMed]
2. McCollum, L.E.; Das, S.R.; Xie, L.; de Flores, R.; Wang, J.; Xie, S.X.; Wisse, L.E.M.; Yushkevich, P.A.; Wolk, D.A. Oh brother, where art tau? Amyloid, neurodegeneration, and cognitive decline without elevated tau. *NeuroImage Clin.* **2021**, *31*, 102717. [CrossRef] [PubMed]
3. Betthauser, T.J.; Koscik, R.L.; Jonaitis, E.M.; Allison, S.L.; Cody, K.A.; Erickson, C.M.; Rowley, H.A.; Stone, C.K.; Mueller, K.D.; Clark, L.R.; et al. Amyloid and tau imaging biomarkers explain cognitive decline from late middle-age. *Brain* **2020**, *143*, 320–335. [CrossRef] [PubMed]
4. Ossenkoppele, R.; Smith, R.; Mattsson-Carlgren, N.; Groot, C.; Leuzy, A.; Strandberg, O.; Palmqvist, S.; Olsson, T.; Jogi, J.; Stormrud, E.; et al. Accuracy of Tau Positron Emission Tomography as a Prognostic Marker in Preclinical and Prodromal Alzheimer Disease: A Head-to-Head Comparison Against Amyloid Positron Emission Tomography and Magnetic Resonance Imaging. *JAMA Neurol.* **2021**, *78*, 961–971. [CrossRef]
5. Buckley, R.F.; Hanseeuw, B.; Schultz, A.P.; Vannini, P.; Aghjayan, S.L.; Properzi, M.J.; Jackson, J.D.; Mormino, E.C.; Rentz, D.M.; Sperling, R.A.; et al. Region-Specific Association of Subjective Cognitive Decline with Tauopathy Independent of Global β-Amyloid Burden. *JAMA Neurol.* **2017**, *74*, 1455–1463. [CrossRef] [PubMed]
6. Maschio, C.; Ni, R. Amyloid and Tau Positron Emission Tomography Imaging in Alzheimer's Disease and Other Tauopathies. *Front. Aging Neurosci.* **2022**, *14*, 838034. [CrossRef]
7. Devous Sr., M.D.; Fleisher, A.S.; Pontecorvo, M.J.; Lu, M.; Siderowf, A.; Navitsky, M.; Kennedy, I.; Southekal, S.; Harris, T.S.; Mintun, M.A. Relationships Between Cognition and Neuropathological Tau in Alzheimer's Disease Assessed by 18F Flortaucipir PET. *J. Alzheimer's Dis.* **2021**, *80*, 1091–1104. [CrossRef]
8. Kroth, H.; Oden, F.; Molette, J.; Schieferstein, H.; Capotosti, F.; Mueller, A.; Berndt, M.; Schmitt-Willich, H.; Darmency, V.; Gabellieri, E.; et al. Discovery and preclinical characterization of [18F]PI-2620, a next-generation tau PET tracer for the assessment of tau pathology in Alzheimer's disease and other tauopathies. *Eur. J. Nucl. Med. Mol. Imaging* **2019**, *46*, 2178–2189. [CrossRef]
9. Shi, Y.; Murzin, A.G.; Falcon, B.; Epstein, A.; Machin, J.; Tempest, P.; Newell, K.L.; Vidal, R.; Garringer, H.J.; Sahara, N.; et al. Cryo-EM structures of tau filaments from Alzheimer's disease with PET ligand APN-1607. *Acta Neuropathol.* **2021**, *141*, 697–708. [CrossRef]
10. Botha, H.; Mantyh, W.G.; Graff-Radford, J.; Machulda, M.M.; Przybelski, S.A.; Wiste, H.J.; Senjem, M.L.; Parisi, J.E.; Petersen, R.C.; Murray, M.E.; et al. Tau-negative amnestic dementia masquerading as Alzheimer disease dementia. *Neurology* **2018**, *90*, e940–e946. [CrossRef]

11. Whitwell, J.L.; Martin, P.; Radford, J.G.; Machulda, M.M.; Senjem, M.L.; Schwarz, C.G.; Weigand, S.D.; Spychalla, A.J.; Drubach, D.A.; Jack, C.R.; et al. The role of age on tau PET uptake and gray matter atrophy in atypical Alzheimer's disease. *Alzheimer's Dement.* **2019**, *15*, 675–685. [CrossRef] [PubMed]
12. Guo, T.; Landau, S.M.; Jagust, W.J. Age, vascular disease, and Alzheimer's disease pathologies in amyloid negative elderly adults. *Alzheimer's Res. Ther.* **2021**, *13*, 174. [CrossRef] [PubMed]
13. Wegmann, S.; Bennett, R.E.; Delorme, L.; Robbins, A.B.; Hu, M.; McKenzie, D.; Kirk, M.J.; Schiantarelli, J.; Tunio, N.; Amaral, A.C.; et al. Experimental evidence for the age dependence of tau protein spread in the brain. *Sci. Adv.* **2019**, *5*, w6404. [CrossRef]
14. Mayerhoefer, M.E.; Materka, A.; Langs, G.; Haggstrom, I.; Szczypinski, P.; Gibbs, P.; Cook, G. Introduction to Radiomics. *J. Nucl. Med.* **2020**, *61*, 488–495. [CrossRef] [PubMed]
15. Jiang, J.; Zhang, J.; Li, Z.; Li, L.; Huang, B. Using Deep Learning Radiomics to Distinguish Cognitively Normal Adults at Risk of Alzheimer's Disease from Normal Control: An Exploratory Study Based on Structural MRI. *Front. Med.* **2022**, *9*, 894726. [CrossRef] [PubMed]
16. Alongi, P.; Laudicella, R.; Panasiti, F.; Stefano, A.; Comelli, A.; Giaccone, P.; Arnone, A.; Minutoli, F.; Quartuccio, N.; Cupidi, C.; et al. Radiomics Analysis of Brain [18F]FDG PET/CT to Predict Alzheimer's Disease in Patients with Amyloid PET Positivity: A Preliminary Report on the Application of SPM Cortical Segmentation, Pyradiomics and Machine-Learning Analysis. *Diagnostics* **2022**, *12*, 933. [CrossRef] [PubMed]
17. Lin, H.; Jiang, J.; Li, Z.; Sheng, C.; Du, W.; Li, X.; Han, Y. Identification of subjective cognitive decline due to Alzheimer's disease using multimodal MRI combining with machine learning. *Cereb. Cortex* **2022**, *33*, 557–566. [CrossRef]
18. Li, Y.; Jiang, J.; Lu, J.; Jiang, J.; Zhang, H.; Zuo, C. Radiomics: A novel feature extraction method for brain neuron degeneration disease using18F-FDG PET imaging and its implementation for Alzheimer's disease and mild cognitive impairment. *Ther. Adv. Neurol. Disord.* **2019**, *12*, 1160684164. [CrossRef]
19. La Joie, R.; Visani, A.V.; Lesman-Segev, O.H.; Baker, S.L.; Edwards, L.; Iaccarino, L.; Soleimani-Meigooni, D.N.; Mellinger, T.; Janabi, M.; Miller, Z.A.; et al. Association of APOE4 and Clinical Variability in Alzheimer Disease with the Pattern of Tau- and Amyloid-PET. *Neurology* **2021**, *96*, e650–e661. [CrossRef]
20. Durairajan, S.S.K.; Selvarasu, K.; Bera, M.R.; Rajaram, K.; Iyaswamy, A.; Li, M. Alzheimer's Disease and other Tauopathies: Exploring Efficacy of Medicinal Plant-derived Compounds in Alleviating Tau-mediated Neurodegeneration. *Curr. Mol. Pharm.* **2022**, *15*, 361. [CrossRef]
21. McKhann, G.M.; Knopman, D.S.; Chertkow, H.; Hyman, B.T.; Jack, C.R., Jr.; Kawas, C.H.; Klunk, W.E.; Koroshetz, W.J.; Manly, J.J.; Mayeux, R.; et al. The diagnosis of dementia due to Alzheimer's disease: Recommendations from the National Institute on Aging-Alzheimer's Association workgroups on diagnostic guidelines for Alzheimer's disease. *Alzheimer's Dement.* **2011**, *7*, 263–269. [CrossRef] [PubMed]
22. Albert, M.S.; DeKosky, S.T.; Dickson, D.; Dubois, B.; Feldman, H.H.; Fox, N.C.; Gamst, A.; Holtzman, D.M.; Jagust, W.J.; Petersen, R.C.; et al. The diagnosis of mild cognitive impairment due to Alzheimer's disease: Recommendations from the National Institute on Aging-Alzheimer's Association workgroups on diagnostic guidelines for Alzheimer's disease. *Alzheimer's Dement.* **2011**, *7*, 270–279. [CrossRef] [PubMed]
23. Liu, F.T.; Li, X.Y.; Lu, J.Y.; Wu, P.; Li, L.; Liang, X.N.; Ju, Z.Z.; Jiao, F.Y.; Chen, M.J.; Ge, J.J.; et al. 18F-FlorzolotauTau Positron Emission Tomography Imaging in Patients with Multiple SystemAtrophy–Parkinsonian Subtype. *Mov. Disord.* **2022**, *37*, 1915–1923. [CrossRef] [PubMed]
24. Hsu, J.; Lin, K.; Hsiao, I.; Huang, K.; Liu, C.; Wu, H.; Weng, Y.; Huang, C.; Chang, C.; Yen, T.; et al. The Imaging Features and Clinical Associations of a Novel Tau PET Tracer—18F-APN1607 in Alzheimer Disease. *Clin. Nucl. Med.* **2020**, *45*, 747–756. [CrossRef] [PubMed]
25. Devous, M.D.; Joshi, A.D.; Navitsky, M.; Southekal, S.; Pontecorvo, M.J.; Shen, H.; Lu, M.; Shankle, W.R.; Seibyl, J.P.; Marek, K.; et al. Test-Retest Reproducibility for the Tau PET Imaging Agent Flortaucipir F 18. *J. Nucl. Med.* **2018**, *59*, 937–943. [CrossRef]
26. Vallières, M.; Freeman, C.R.; Skamene, S.R.; El Naqa, I. A radiomics model from joint FDG-PET and MRI texture features for the prediction of lung metastases in soft-tissue sarcomas of the extremities. *Phys. Med. Biol.* **2015**, *60*, 5471–5496. [CrossRef]
27. Feng, Q.; Ding, Z. MRI Radiomics Classification and Prediction in Alzheimer's Disease and Mild Cognitive Impairment: A Review. *Curr. Alzheimer Res.* **2020**, *17*, 297–309. [CrossRef]
28. Won, S.Y.; Park, Y.W.; Park, M.; Ahn, S.S.; Kim, J.; Lee, S. Quality Reporting of Radiomics Analysis in Mild Cognitive Impairment and Alzheimer's Disease: A Roadmap for Moving Forward. *Korean J. Radiol.* **2020**, *21*, 1345–1354. [CrossRef]
29. Feng, Q.; Niu, J.; Wang, L.; Pang, P.; Wang, M.; Liao, Z.; Song, Q.; Jiang, H.; Ding, Z. Comprehensive classification models based on amygdala radiomic features for Alzheimer's disease and mild cognitive impairment. *Brain Imaging Behav.* **2021**, *15*, 2377–2386. [CrossRef]
30. Du, Y.; Zhang, S.; Fang, Y.; Qiu, Q.; Zhao, L.; Wei, W.; Tang, Y.; Li, X. Radiomic Features of the Hippocampus for Diagnosing Early-Onset and Late-Onset Alzheimer's Disease. *Front. Aging Neurosci.* **2022**, *13*, 789099. [CrossRef]
31. Ding, Y.; Zhao, K.; Che, T.; Du, K.; Sun, H.; Liu, S.; Zheng, Y.; Li, S.; Liu, B.; Liu, Y. Quantitative Radiomic Features as New Biomarkers for Alzheimer's Disease: An Amyloid PET Study. *Cereb. Cortex* **2021**, *31*, 3950–3961. [CrossRef] [PubMed]
32. Zhang, H.; Wang, M.; Lu, J.; Bao, W.; Li, L.; Jiang, J.; Zuo, C. Parametric Estimation of Reference Signal Intensity for Semi-Quantification of Tau Deposition: A Flortaucipir and [18F]-APN-1607 Study. *Front. Neurosci.* **2021**, *15*, 598234. [CrossRef] [PubMed]

33. Pinto, T.C.C.; Machado, L.; Bulgacov, T.M.; Rodrigues-Júnior, A.L.; Costa, M.L.G.; Ximenes, R.C.C.; Sougey, E.B. Is the Montreal Cognitive Assessment (MoCA) screening superior to the Mini-Mental State Examination (MMSE) in the detection of mild cognitive impairment (MCI) and Alzheimer's Disease (AD) in the elderly? *Int. Psychogeriatr.* **2019**, *31*, 491–504. [CrossRef] [PubMed]
34. Huang, K.; Lin, Y.; Yang, L.; Wang, Y.; Cai, S.; Pang, L.; Wu, X.; Huang, L. A multipredictor model to predict the conversion of mild cognitive impairment to Alzheimer's disease by using a predictive nomogram. *Neuropsychopharmacology* **2020**, *45*, 358–366. [CrossRef] [PubMed]
35. Abner, E.L.; Kryscio, R.J.; Schmitt, F.A.; Fardo, D.W.; Moga, D.C.; Ighodaro, E.T.; Jicha, G.A.; Yu, L.; Dodge, H.H.; Xiong, C.; et al. Outcomes after diagnosis of mild cognitive impairment in a large autopsy series. *Ann. Neurol.* **2017**, *81*, 549–559. [CrossRef] [PubMed]
36. Josephs, K.A.; Weigand, S.D.; Whitwell, J.L. Characterizing Amyloid-Positive Individuals with Normal Tau PET Levels After 5 Years. *Neurology* **2022**, *98*, e2282–e2292. [CrossRef] [PubMed]
37. Ren, D.; Lopez, O.L.; Lingler, J.H.; Conley, Y. The Effect of the APOE $\varepsilon 2\varepsilon 4$ Genotype on the Development of Alzheimer's Disease (AD) and Mild Cognitive Impairment (MCI) in Non-Latino Whites. *J. Am. Geriatr. Soc.* **2020**, *68*, 1044–1049. [CrossRef]
38. Yan, S.; Zheng, C.; Paranjpe, M.D.; Li, Y.; Li, W.; Wang, X.; Benzinger, T.L.S.; Lu, J.; Zhou, Y. Sex modifies APOE $\varepsilon 4$ dose effect on brain tau deposition in cognitively impaired individuals. *Brain* **2021**, *144*, 3201–3211. [CrossRef]
39. Safieh, M.; Korczyn, A.D.; Michaelson, D.M. ApoE4: An emerging therapeutic target for Alzheimer's disease. *BMC Med.* **2019**, *17*, 64. [CrossRef]
40. Jellinger, K.A. Recent update on the heterogeneity of the Alzheimer's disease spectrum. *J. Neural Transm.* **2022**, *129*, 1–24. [CrossRef]

Disclaimer/Publisher's Note: The statements, opinions and data contained in all publications are solely those of the individual author(s) and contributor(s) and not of MDPI and/or the editor(s). MDPI and/or the editor(s) disclaim responsibility for any injury to people or property resulting from any ideas, methods, instructions or products referred to in the content.

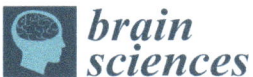

Article

Development of a Machine Learning Model to Discriminate Mild Cognitive Impairment Subjects from Normal Controls in Community Screening

Juanjuan Jiang [1], Jieming Zhang [1], Chenyang Li [2], Zhihua Yu [3], Zhuangzhi Yan [2,*] and Jiehui Jiang [2]

1 School of Communication and Information Engineering, Shanghai University, Shanghai 200444, China
2 Institute of Biomedical Engineering, School of Life Science, Shanghai University, Shanghai 200444, China
3 Shanghai Geriatric Institute of Chinese Medicine, Shanghai University of Traditional Chinese Medicine, Shanghai 200031, China
* Correspondence: zzyan@shu.edu.cn

Abstract: Background: Mild cognitive impairment (MCI) is a transitional stage between normal aging and probable Alzheimer's disease. It is of great value to screen for MCI in the community. A novel machine learning (ML) model is composed of electroencephalography (EEG), eye tracking (ET), and neuropsychological assessments. This study has been proposed to identify MCI subjects from normal controls (NC). **Methods**: Two cohorts were used in this study. Cohort 1 as the training and validation group, includes184 MCI patients and 152 NC subjects. Cohort 2 as an independent test group, includes 44 MCI and 48 NC individuals. EEG, ET, Neuropsychological Tests Battery (NTB), and clinical variables with age, gender, educational level, MoCA-B, and ACE-R were selected for all subjects. Receiver operating characteristic (ROC) curves were adopted to evaluate the capabilities of this tool to classify MCI from NC. The clinical model, the EEG and ET model, and the neuropsychological model were compared. **Results**: We found that the classification accuracy of the proposed model achieved 84.5 ± 4.43% and 88.8 ± 3.59% in Cohort 1 and Cohort 2, respectively. The area under curve (AUC) of the proposed tool achieved 0.941 (0.893–0.982) in Cohort 1 and 0.966 (0.921–0.988) in Cohort 2, respectively. **Conclusions**: The proposed model incorporation of EEG, ET, and neuropsychological assessments yielded excellent classification performances, suggesting its potential for future application in cognitive decline prediction.

Keywords: mild cognitive impairment; neuropsychological tests battery; machine learning; screening tool

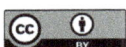

1. Introduction

Alzheimer's disease (AD) is the most common neurodegenerative brain disease that affects 50–70% of patients with cognitive impairments over the age of 65 [1]. AD pathology leads to an irreversible deterioration in cognitive functions such as loss of memory, executive dysfunction, and attention disorders [2–4]. Mild cognitive impairment (MCI) refers to the intermediate period between the typical cognitive decline of normal aging and the more severe decline associated with dementia (e.g., AD) [5–7]. Because of the irreversibility of AD, it is of great value to screen MCI subjects at the community level [5,8,9].

Currently, biochemical tests (e.g., Cerebrospinal Fluid and Blood) and neuroimaging tests (e.g., Magnetic Resonance Imaging,) were considered efficient screening tools for MCI [10–12]. However, these techniques were usually invasive and expensive, restricting large-scale screening applications in the community [13,14]. Therefore, an effective and low-cost detectable approach to cognitive decline in MCI is urgently required.

Recently, MCI screening has attracted immersive interests. A Neuropsychological Tests Battery (NTB) is well recognized in the diagnostic pipelines of preclinical AD [15]. Multiple preclinical neuropsychological measures significantly predicted progression to

AD from MCI and detected changes in patients in verbal and visual memory, visuospatial processing, error control, and subjective neuropsychological complaints [16]. Paul et. al. confirmed that neuropsychological tests quick-MCI to assess cognitive status in 3–5 min and can discriminate MCI accurately in primary care [17]. Neuropsychological tests were clearly appropriate for MCI community screening, as are emerging cognitive assessments such as electroencephalogram (EEG) and eye tracking (ET) to monitor cognitive function. Murty et al. found that stimulus-induced gamma rhythms from EEG were significantly lower in MCI/AD subjects compared to their age- and gender-matched controls, suggesting that gamma of EEG could be used as a potential screening tool for MCI or AD in humans [18]. Oyama et al. developed a brief cognitive assessment utilizing an eye-tracking technology that can enable quantitative scoring and the sensitive detection of cognitive impairment in patients with mild cognitive impairment and dementia [19]. Nie et al. found that eye movement parameters are stable indicators to distinguish patients with MCI and cognitively normal subjects and are not affected by different testing versions and numbers [20]. The incorporation of neuropsychological tests and physiological measurements warrants further study as a practical and cost-effective method for wide-scale screening for identifying older adults who may be at risk for pathological cognitive decline. Neuropsychological tests might be limited in their effectiveness in MCI screening while acknowledging that neuropsychological tests are inadequate for making a definitive diagnosis. To increase the precision and sensitivity of MCI screening, several researchers incorporated NTB into objective physiological measures, such as prefrontal EEG [21] and ET [22]. For instance, our previous work validated the feasibility of physiological measures using EEG and ET in distinguishing MCI from HC, with a classification accuracy of 81.5% [23].

In addition, with the development of artificial intelligence techniques, machine learning (ML) methods have been widely used for the differential diagnosis of MCI [15,23–25]. For example, Lin et al. developed non-invasive clinical variables and ML classifiers, including Support Vector Machine (SVM), Logistic Regression (LR), and Random Forest (RF), to achieve over 75% classification accuracy to classify subjects who converted to MCI from normal within four years [25]. Yim et al. proposed a ML algorithm to identify cognitive dysfunction based on neuropsychological tests including the Montreal Cognitive Assessment (MoCA). The results showed a good classification performance between cognitive impairment and normal subjects [15]. However, there were few models using neuropsychological tests, physiological tests, and ML algorithms in the previous studies.

This study aims to propose and validate a novel and low-cost screening model consisting of neuropsychological tests, physiological tests, and ML algorithms. Importantly, to evaluate the robustness of the model, two independent cohorts were used in this study.

2. MCI Prediction Algorithms

Figure 1 shows the flowchart of the proposed model, which was composed of four steps: data collection, data preprocessing, feature extraction and selection, and classification based on ML classifiers. These steps were described in detail as the following:

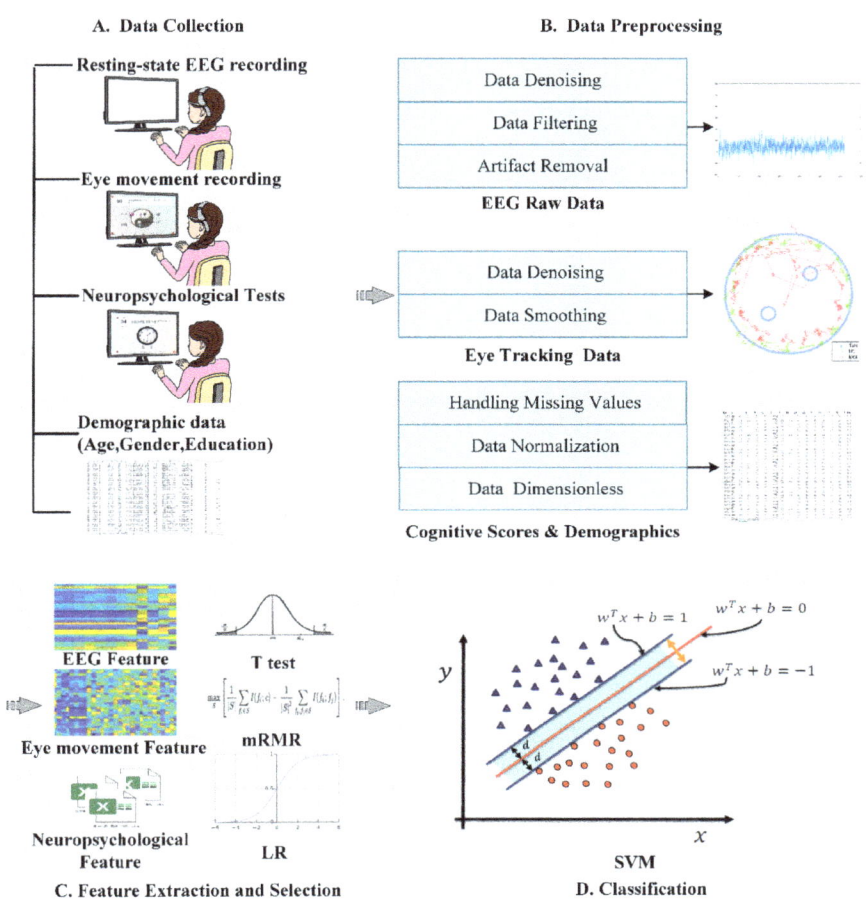

Figure 1. The flowchart of the proposed model.

2.1. Data Collection

EEG, ET, neuropsychological test (Table S1), and demographic data (age, gender, and education) were selected as the inputs of the model. Details of the data collection step were described in our previous study [23] and provided in the Figure S1 of Supplementary Material.

2.2. Data Preprocessing

This model included an automatic data preprocessing step for EEG, ET, and NTB.

2.2.1. EEG Preprocessing

Invalid EEG data was first removed according to whether the EEG electrode was offset. Next, the power frequency noise, electromyogram signal, electrocardiogram signal, and other external noises were removed using a band stop filter and a band pass filter. Simple second-order Butterworth filtering was applied with a passband of 0.5–30 Hz. Finally, we overlapped 60% of the EEG data by applying a 5 s moving window, providing 15 overlapping segments for each subject. The EEG signal was preprocessing using EEGLAB toolbox implemented in MATLAB 2018a (Math Works Inc., Sherborn, MA, USA).

2.2.2. ET Preprocessing

First, excessive noise from ET data was eliminated. Next, the gaze position signal was normalized to the display coordinates to avoid the interpolation bias. Finally, a low pass Butterworth filter with a cut-off frequency of 5 Hz was implemented in MATLAB 2018a (Math Works Inc., Sherborn, MA, USA).

2.2.3. NTB Data Preprocessing

NTB data were cleaned, and all abnormal values were eliminated. Finally, neuropsychological test scores were normalized into 0–1.

2.3. Feature Extraction

2.3.1. EEG Data

Frequency-domain and spectral-domain features of the EEG signal were extracted. A Fourier transform of the autocorrelation function was employed to transform the EEG signal from time-domain to frequency-domain to get the power spectral density. Four EEG frequency bands (delta 0.5–4 Hz, theta 4–8 Hz, alpha 8–13 Hz, and beta 13–30 Hz) were filtered in this study. The power spectrum of each frequency band and specific spectral power ratios like the alpha/theta power ratio was computed. The extracted linear features of the EEG were consistent with our preliminary work [23]. Nonlinear features of the EEG, including approximate entropy (ApEn) [26], Multiscale entropy (MsEn) [27], and Lempel Ziv complexity (LZC) were calculated [28]. The calculation formulas of the EEG features were described in the section of Feature extraction and selection of Supplementary Material.

2.3.2. ET Data

ET data was divided into saccade data and gaze data. The association of gazes and saccades with specific regions on visual stimuli was examined. Then, visual scan parameters such as blink frequency, blink time, fixation time, and sustained attention duration were calculated. The nonlinear features of ET were extracted by LZC.

2.3.3. NTB Data

NTB data, which are numerical, included subtest scores, total test scores, and response time. Meaningful numerical features were subsequently converted to z-scores using Z transformation.

2.4. Feature Selection

The Minimum Redundancy-Maximum Relevance (MRMR) algorithm was used for feature selection [29]. In the MRMR algorithm, the correlation between different feature subsets is modeled as:

$$\Theta = \frac{1}{|\Omega|} \sum_{m} \sum_{f_i \in \Omega} M(f_i, m) \quad (1)$$

where the feature subset Ω is from the feature set F and $F = \{f_1, \ldots, f_D\}$. In this tool, $m = \{+1, -1\}$ represents HC and MCI respectively and M is the mutual information between the feature subset and the target classes which is given by

$$M(X, Y) = \sum_{X} \sum_{Y} p(X, Y) \log_2 \left(\frac{p(X, Y)}{p(X)p(Y)} \right) \quad (2)$$

where $p(X)$, $p(Y)$, $p(X, Y)$ are the marginal probability distributions and joint probability distributions of variable X, Y respectively. Clearly, the mutual information comes to zero when $p(X, Y) = p(X)p(Y)$, which states that the feature is independent with the target classes.

The redundancy between the feature f_i and other features can be modeled as:

$$\Delta_{\Omega,f_i} = \frac{1}{|\Omega|^2} \sum_{f_j \subset \Omega, f_i \neq f_j} M(f_i, f_j) \tag{3}$$

Thus, the feature meeting the minimum redundancy-maximum correlation principle can be obtained via:

$$f_i^* = \underset{f_i \subset \Omega}{\operatorname{argmax}} \frac{\Theta}{\Delta_{\Omega,f_i}} \tag{4}$$

In the above equation, the optimal features can be obtained by maximizing the correlation between the features and the target classification and minimizing the redundancy between the features. By performing similar operations on different feature subsets, multiple optimal features can be found to reduce the complexity and improve the algorithm decision performance.

2.5. Classification

A support vector machine (SVM) was used as the ML classifier with Anaconda Spyder 3.7 (Anaconda Inc., Austin, TX, USA). As a classic supervised learning method, SVM has been widely used in statistical classification and regression analysis due to its ability to map vectors linearly to a higher dimensional space that creates a maximum margin hyperplane to achieve high classification performance.

$$w^T x + b = 0 \tag{5}$$

Support vectors maximize the margin of the classifier by changing the position and orientation of the hyperplane. Kernel functions of SVM or "kernel trick" by SVM were applied to remedy the issue that the points are not separable linearly due to the position of the data. Kernel trick involves the transformation of the existing algorithm from a lower-dimensional data set to a higher one. The amount of information remains the same, but in this higher dimensional space, it is possible to create a linear classifier. Several K kernels are assigned to each point which then helps determine the best fit hyperplane for the newly transformed feature space. With enough K functions, it is possible to get precise separation.

Linear SVM classifier with hard margin:

$$W(\alpha) = -\sum_{i=1}^{l} \alpha_i + \frac{1}{2} \sum_{i=1}^{l} \sum_{j=1}^{l} y_i y_j \alpha_i \alpha_j X_i X_j \tag{6}$$

Kernel trick equation minimizing W subject to:

$$\sum_{i=1}^{l} y_i \alpha_i = 0 \qquad 0 \leq \alpha_i \leq C \tag{7}$$

3. Materials and Methods

3.1. Subjects

We recruited two cohorts for this study. Cohort 1 was composed of 336 subjects from four communities in Jiading district, Shanghai, China, including 152 MCI patients and 184 normal controls (NC) subjects. Cohort 2 was composed of 44 MCI patients and 48 NC subjects from one community in Baoshan district, Shanghai, China. All subjects also underwent a battery of cognitive evaluations, including Addenbrooke's Cognitive Examination-revised (ACE-R) and Montreal cognitive assessment-basic (MoCA-B). The permission of MoCA-B in the study was received via https://www.mocatest.org/permission (accessed on 28 June 2017).

All subjects signed an informed consent before the examinations. This study has been approved by the ethics committee of Long Hua Hospital in Shanghai University of Traditional Chinese Medicine (Ethical number: 2017LCSY345) and conducted in accordance with the principles of the Declaration of Helsinki. In this study, Cohort 1 was used as the training and validation group to train the SVM classifier. Cohort 2 was used as an independent test group to verify the robustness of the classification results.

MCI was defined by an actuarial neuropsychological strategy proposed by Jak and Bondi [30], subjects were considered to have MCI if they met any of the following three criteria and neglected to meet the criteria for dementia. The inclusion criteria for MCI were as follows [31,32]: (1) right-handed, and Mandarin-speaking subjects; (2) a subjective memory complaint; (3) memory impairment relative to age and education-matched healthy elderly individuals confirmed by performance on neuropsychological assessments (below 1.5 standard deviations); (4) intact general cognitive function confirmed by MoCA-B scores ≥ 26; (5) intact activities of daily living; and (6) without dementia confirmed by a physician.

Exclusion criteria of MCI were as follows: (1) other neurological diseases including cerebrovascular disease, brain trauma, Parkinson's syndrome, brain tumor, and epilepsy; (2) current major psychiatric disease such as severe depression and anxiety; (3) other neurological conditions that could cause cognitive decline (e.g., brain tumors, Parkinson's disease, encephalitis, or epilepsy) rather than AD spectrum disorders; (4) systemic diseases that may lead to cognitive decline (thyroid dysfunction, severe anemia, syphilis, or HIV, etc.); (5) other conditions such as a history of CO poisoning and general anesthesia; (6) severe visual or hearing impairment; (7) contraindication for MRI.

The inclusion criteria for NC included the following: (1) no subjective or informant-reported memory decline; (2) non-clinical depression (Geriatric Depression Scale scores < 6); (3) normal age-adjusted, gender-adjusted, and education-adjusted performance on standardized cognitive tests.

3.2. Data Acquisition

All data were selected from 1 September 2017 to 31 August 2018 in the communities, Shanghai, China. The data selection protocol has been introduced in the Supplementary Material.

3.3. Validation Experiments for Optimal Parameters of the Classifier

We adjusted the hyper-parameters for the SVM classifier such as kernel function, penalty factor C, and coefficient of kernel function gamma with good classification performance by 5-fold cross-validation. Different kernels, including linear, polynomial, and RBF were compared in this study. Cohort 1 was used to train these parameters.

3.4. Discriminative Analysis

The classification results from four models were compared by using the SVM classifier, including (1) the clinical model (clinical variables including age, gender, educational level, MoCA-B, ACE-R), (2) the single neuropsychological test model (20 subtests of NTB showed in the Supplementary Material), (3) the single physiological test model (EEG and ET), and (4) the proposed tool model. We used the 5-fold cross-validation method to calculate the classification results.

3.5. Statistical Analysis

Differences in demographic and cognitive performance between the NC group and the MCI group were evaluated by two sample t-tests or chi-square (χ^2) tests of Statistical Package V24 for Social Sciences (SPSS Inc., Chicago, IL, USA). The significance level was set as $p < 0.05$. Receiver operating characteristic (ROC) curves were used to evaluate the capabilities of the tool in distinguishing MCI from NC. The areas under the curves (AUCs) with 95% confidence intervals (CIs) were calculated.

4. Results

4.1. Demographic and Clinical Characteristics

The detailed demographic and clinical characteristics were reported in Table 1. The results showed that the scores of MoCA-B and ACE-R from MCI patients were significantly lower than NC's scores ($p < 0.001$, two-sample t-test). There were no significant differences in age ($p = 0.875$; two-sample t-test), gender ($p = 0.541$; chi-square test) or years of education ($p = 0.071$; Wilcoxon rank-sum test) of cohort 1. There were no significant differences in age ($p = 0.783$; two-sample t-test), gender ($p = 0.492$; chi-square test) or years of education ($p = 0.068$; Wilcoxon rank-sum test) of cohort 2 either.

Table 1. Demographic and clinical characteristics of subjects.

	Cohort 1			Cohort 2		
	NC (184)	MCI (152)	p Value	NC (48)	MCI (44)	p Value
Age (years)	71.7 ± 4.66	71.6 ± 4.15	0.875 [b]	69.3 ± 17.0	76.5 ± 11.3	0.783 [b]
Education (years)	9.36 ± 3.47	8.16 ± 3.74	0.541 [a]	13.0 ± 3.87	10.8 ± 5.66	0.492 [a]
Gender (male/female)	101/83	78/74	0.071 [c]	18/30	16/28	0.068 [c]
MoCA-B	28.3 ± 0.95	23.2 ± 3.40	<0.001 [b] *	23.8 ± 3.28	16.4 ± 3.84	<0.001 [b] *
ACE-R	72.1 ± 7.79	63.7 ± 8.53	<0.001 [b] *	71.0 ± 24.9	64.2 ± 8.28	<0.001 [b] *

Note: Data are presented as mean ± standard deviation. * Indicates a statistical difference between groups, $p < 0.05$; [a]: the p value was obtained by χ2 test, [b]: the p value was obtained by two-sample t tests, [c]: the p value was obtained by Wilcoxon rank-sum test. Abbreviations: NC, normal control; MCI, Mild Cognitive Impairment; MoCA-B, Montreal cognitive assessment-basic; ACE-R, Addenbrooke's Cognitive Examination Revised.

4.2. Validation Experiments for Optimal Parameters of Classifier

The best classification performance was obtained under the specific parameters (C = 1.1, GAMMA = 0.001) while the kernel function was set to RBF. Table 2 shows the detailed performance of different kernel functions and corresponding parameters.

Table 2. The optimized hyper-parameters of SVM in test dataset.

Kernel Function	C	GAMMA	Accuracy (%)	Sensitivity (%)	Specificity (%)	AUC (95% CI)
Linear	4.0	/	84.3 ± 4.05	83.1 ± 7.70	85.5 ± 4.97	0.906 (0.841–0.969)
Poly	20.0	0.02	78.1 ± 9.90	83.6 ± 10.6	71.3 ± 13.6	0.851 (0.747–0.954)
RBF	**1.1**	**0.001**	**84.5 ± 4.34**	82.4 ± 7.36	**86.5 ± 6.51**	**0.934 (0.878–0.977)**
Sigmoid	17.0	0.01	82.1 ± 6.08	**90.9 ± 8.13**	71.3 ± 11.7	0.851 (0.838–0.964)

C represents the regularization coefficient, gamma represents the kernel function coefficient, AUC represents the area under the ROC curve, the bold part in the table is the optimal value of each column, and the values in the table are the mean and standard deviation after five cross-validations.

4.3. Discriminative Analysis

Tables 3 and 4 showed comparison results of four models in Cohort 1 and 2, respectively. Classification results showed that the performance of the proposed tool was better than other models (Accuracy: 84.5 ± 4.43%; Sensitivity: 81.9 ± 7.88%; Specificity: 86.8 ± 6.19%; AUC: 0.942 (0.893–0.982)) in Cohort 1. Classification results also showed that the performance of the proposed tool was better than other models (Accuracy: 88.8 ± 3.59%; Sensitivity: 86.2 ± 6.46%; Specificity: 91.0 ± 5.39%; AUC: 0.966 (0.921–0.988)) in Cohort 2. Figures 2 and 3 showed the ROC results of the four models in both cohorts.

Table 3. The classification results of four models in cohort 1.

Comparative Model	Accuracy (%)	Sensitivity (%)	Specificity (%)	AUC (95% CI)
The clinical model	62.6 ± 5.19	54.7 ± 6.81	71.4 ± 5.56	0.653 (0.541–0.783)
Single neuropsychological test model	75.6 ± 4.60	55.7 ± 8.15	71.2 ± 4.72	0.8014 (0.700–0.885)
Single physiological test model	81.4 ± 4.66	72.1 ± 8.25	89.2 ± 5.42	0.9045 (0.819–0.961)
The proposed tool model	84.5 ± 4.43	81.9 ± 7.88	86.8 ± 6.19	0.9415 (0.893–0.982)

Table 4. The classification results of four models in cohort 2.

Comparative Model	Accuracy (%)	Sensitivity (%)	Specificity (%)	AUC (95% CI)
The clinical model	65.7 ± 4.93	43.3 ± 10.6	90.1 ± 7.94	0.660 (0.543–0.789)
Single neuropsychological test model	75.0 ± 5.22	54.1 ± 8.63	91.5 ± 4.73	0.803 (0.681–0.889)
Single physiological test model	87.0 ± 4.27	82.4 ± 7.94	90.6 ± 5.05	0.937 (0.867–0.985)
The proposed tool model	88.8 ± 3.59	86.2 ± 6.46	91.0 ± 5.39	0.966 (0.921–0.988)

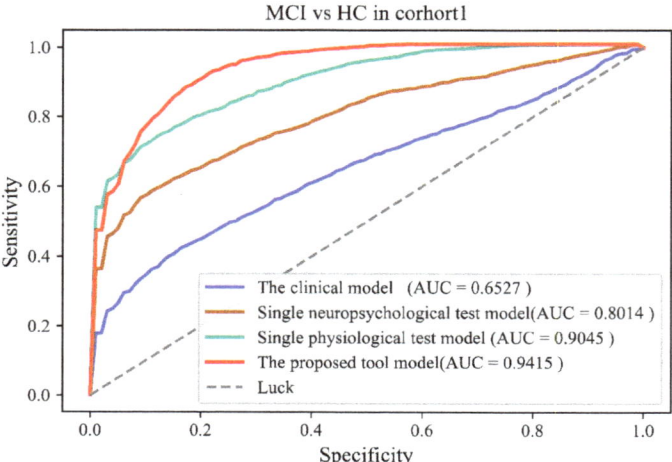

Figure 2. The receiver operating curves of four models in cohort 1.

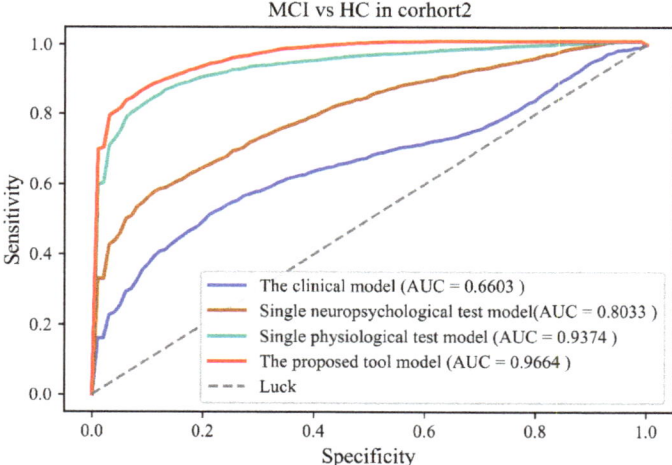

Figure 3. The receiver operating curves of four models in cohort 2.

5. Discussion

Cognitive decline remains highly underdiagnosed in the community despite extensive efforts to find novel approaches to detect MCI and find objective screening methods for cognitive decline could improve early MCI diagnosis. MCI screening in the community has become a hot topic nowadays. In light of their excellent performance in detecting a cognitive decline in MCI patients, multimodal detection approaches have been commonly used in computer-aided disease diagnostic fields of community screening. In this study, we proposed a ML model based on EEG, eye movement, and neuropsychological tests for MCI screening at the community level. In contrast to other traditional models, such as the EEG-based model, ET-based model, and NTB-based model, the classification results of our model outperformed other traditional models.

So far, a lot of studies have focused on the classification of NC and MCI by using machine learning models for screening in primary care. For instance, Siuly et al. performed a Piecewise Aggregate Approximation (PAA) technique for compressing massive volumes of EEG data for reliable analysis and developed a model based on Extreme Learning Machine (ELM) with permutation entropy (PE) and auto-regressive (AR) model features to achieve the highest MCI classification accuracy (98.8%) [33]; Lagun et al. applied a SVM based machine learning model to reach the accuracy of 87% to detect MCI by modeling eye movement characteristics such as fixations, saccades, and refixations during the Visual Paired Comparison (VPC) task [34]; Yim et al. developed a screening model based on a gradient boosting (GB) algorithm to identify MCI by neuropsychological test results and reached the classification accuracy of 93.5% [15]; and, Wang et al. developed a Random Forest (RF)-based model to optimize the content of cognitive evaluation and achieved an accuracy of 68% in the classification of MCI and NC [35].

Notably, our classification results were similar to previous studies, indicating the reliability of our results. As shown in Table 5, although previous studies based on EEG analysis performed powerful discrimination for MCI detection (ACC = 98.8% in Siuly's model), it is worth noting that these studies based on expensive and long-term physiological signal collection devices are seldom used in primary care. By contrast, the wearable EEG device used in our approach was more suitable for large-scale MCI screening. In contrast to earlier studies based on ET and NTB, our method achieved better accuracy. Additionally, the advantages of our method were also summarized as follows:

Table 5. The performance of analogous MCI detection methods in the literature.

Detection Tools	Modality	Subject	Method	Classifier	Accuracy
EEG based	Siuly, 2020 [33] EEG (19 Electrodes)	27	EEG features	ELM	98.8%
ET based	Lagun, 2011 [34] ET Test	174	ET features	SVM	87%
Neuropsychological test based	Yim, 2020 [15]	614	The mean total scores of neuropsychological test	GB	93.5%
NTB based	Wang, 2022 [35] Neuropsychological tests battery	241	NTB scores	RF	68%
Proposed Method NTB, EEG and Eye tracking	EEG (1 electrode) & ET & Neuropsychological test battery	336	EEG & ET features & NTB scores	SVM	88.8%

(1) In terms of feature extraction, the linear and nonlinear feature analysis has been successfully used to identify the powerful biomarkers of neurophysiological diseases, such as Alzheimer's disease (AD). In this study, we applied both linear and nonlinear methods to extract EEG and eye movement features. For EEG, complexity analysis as a nonlinear dynamic method can represent the rate of new patterns appearing in a time series, and to a certain extent, details of the signal can be presented in the binarized sequence.

(2) In terms of feature selection and classification, the SVM model was selected. As a ML model, the SVM is suitable for classifying the features obtained from neuropsychological assessments.

(3) In terms of the clinical setting, we depicted a machine learning framework for automated cognitive assessment data analysis for the precise classification of healthy and mild cognitive impairment individuals. Our work opens the possibility for automated assessment of cognitive function in community screening.

Although our proposed method achieved a good classification of screening MCI and NC, several limitations still exist. First, the whole experiment is time-consuming and thus leads to a decrease in the degree of completion and cooperation of patients. Second, the de-noising algorithm may influence the results of feature extraction and classification. Third, the sample size of NC and MCI individuals was limited, and increasing the sample size in future studies should be taken into consideration. Longitudinal imaging studies are still absent. In the subsequent research, ongoing follow-up observational studies of individuals will facilitate the investigation and validation of our results. Finally, SVM was only used as the classifier in this study. If alternative classifiers such as using extreme learning machines or deep learning models were developed, better classification results will be obtained.

6. Conclusions

In this study, an automatic and non-invasive MCI detection model was proposed, which integrated EEG, Eye movement techniques, and a neuropsychological test battery. The results indicated the potential application for MCI detection and guided referral for a more comprehensive evaluation to ultimately facilitate early intervention in primary care.

Supplementary Materials: The following supporting information can be downloaded at: https://www.mdpi.com/article/10.3390/brainsci12091149/s1. Figure S1. Data collection in this study. Table S1. listed neuropsychological Test used in this study.

Author Contributions: Conceptualization, Z.Y. (Zhuangzhi Yan) and J.J. (Jiehui Jiang); methodology, J.J. (Juanjuan Jiang); software, J.Z.; validation, C.L.; formal analysis, J.J. (Juanjuan Jiang); investigation, C.L.; data curation, J.Z.; writing—original draft preparation, J.J. (Juanjuan Jiang); writing—review and editing, J.J. (Juanjuan Jiang); supervision, Z.Y. (Zhihua Yu); project administration, Z.Y. (Zhihua Yu). All authors have read and agreed to the published version of the manuscript.

Funding: This research was funded by Science and Technology Innovation 2030 Major Projects (2022ZD0211600), National Natural Science Foundation of China (Grant 82020108013), and Research project of Shanghai Health Commission (2020YJZX0111).

Institutional Review Board Statement: All procedures performed in studies involving human participants were in accordance with the ethical standards of either the institutional or national research committee and with the 1964 Helsinki Declaration and its later amendments or comparable ethical standards. The study was approved by the Ethics Committee of Long Hua Hospital in Shanghai University of Traditional Chinese Medicine (Ethical number: 2017LCSY345).

Informed Consent Statement: Informed consent was obtained from all subjects involved in the study. Written informed consent has been obtained from the subjects to publish this paper.

Data Availability Statement: The data that support the findings of this study are available from the corresponding author.

Conflicts of Interest: The authors declare no conflict of interest.

References

1. Rocaspana-García, M.; Blanco-Blanco, J.; Arias-Pastor, A.; Gea-Sánchez, M.; Piñol-Ripoll, G.J.P. Study of community-living Alzheimer's patients' adherence to the Mediterranean diet and risks of malnutrition at different disease stages. *PeerJ* **2018**, *6*, e5150. [CrossRef] [PubMed]
2. Jia, L.; Quan, M.; Fu, Y.; Zhao, T.; Li, Y.; Wei, C.; Tang, Y.; Qin, Q.; Wang, F.; Qiao, Y.; et al. Dementia in China: Epidemiology, clinical management, and research advances. *Lancet Neurol.* **2020**, *19*, 81–92. [CrossRef]
3. Jia, L.; Du, Y.; Chu, L.; Zhang, Z.; Li, F.; Lyu, D.; Li, Y.; Li, Y.; Zhu, M.; Jiao, H.; et al. Prevalence, risk factors, and management of dementia and mild cognitive impairment in adults aged 60 years or older in China: A cross-sectional study. *Lancet Public Health* **2020**, *5*, e661–e671. [CrossRef]
4. Petersen, R.C.; Roberts, R.O.; Knopman, D.S.; Boeve, B.F.; Geda, Y.E.; Ivnik, R.J.; Smith, G.E.; Jack, C.R., Jr. Mild cognitive impairment: Ten years later. *Arch. Neurol.* **2009**, *66*, 1447–1455. [CrossRef]
5. Petersen, R.C.; Smith, G.E.; Waring, S.C.; Ivnik, R.J.; Tangalos, E.G.; Kokmen, E. Mild cognitive impairment: Clinical characterization and outcome. *Arch. Neurol.* **1999**, *56*, 303–308. [CrossRef]

6. Wang, M.; Jiang, J.; Yan, Z.; Alberts, I.L.; Ge, J.; Zhang, H.; Zuo, C.; Yu, J.; Rominger, A.; Shi, K.; et al. Individual brain metabolic connectome indicator based on Kullback-Leibler Divergence Similarity Estimation predicts progression from mild cognitive impairment to Alzheimer's dementia. *Eur. J. Nucl. Med. Mol. Imaging* **2020**, *47*, 2753–2764. [CrossRef]
7. Jiang, J.; Sun, X.-M.; Alberts, I.L.; Wang, M.; Rominger, A.; Zuo, C.; Han, Y.; Shi, K.; Initiative, F.T.A.D.N. Using radiomics-based modelling to predict individual progression from mild cognitive impairment to Alzheimer's disease. *Eur. J. Nucl. Med. Mol. Imaging* **2022**, *49*, 2163–2173. [CrossRef]
8. Jack, C.R., Jr.; Bennett, D.A.; Blennow, K.; Carrillo, M.C.; Dunn, B.; Haeberlein, S.B.; Holtzman, D.M.; Jagust, W.; Jessen, F.; Karlawish, J.; et al. NIA-AA Research Framework: Toward a biological definition of Alzheimer's disease. *Alzheimers Dement.* **2018**, *14*, 535–562. [CrossRef]
9. Petersen, R.C.; Yaffe, K. Issues and Questions Surrounding Screening for Cognitive Impairment in Older Patients. *JAMA* **2020**, *323*, 722–724. [CrossRef]
10. Marcucci, V.; Kleiman, J.D. Biomarkers and Their Implications in Alzheimer's Disease: A Literature Review. *Explor. Res. Hypothesis Med.* **2021**, *6*, 164–176. [CrossRef]
11. Chandra, A.; Dervenoulas, G.; Politis, M. Magnetic resonance imaging in Alzheimer's disease and mild cognitive impairment. *J. Neurol.* **2018**, *266*, 1293–1302. [CrossRef] [PubMed]
12. Arbizu, J.; Festari, C.; Altomare, D.; Walker, Z.; Bouwman, F.H.; Rivolta, J.; Orini, S.; Barthel, H.; Agosta, F.; Drzezga, A.; et al. Clinical utility of FDG-PET for the clinical diagnosis in MCI. *Eur. J. Nucl. Med. Mol. Imaging* **2018**, *45*, 1497–1508. [CrossRef] [PubMed]
13. Alberdi, A.; Aztiria, A.; Basarab, A. On the early diagnosis of Alzheimer's Disease from multimodal signals: A survey. *Artif. Intell. Med.* **2016**, *71*, 1–29. [CrossRef] [PubMed]
14. Laske, C.; Sohrabi, H.R.; Frost, S.; Lopez-de-Ipina, K.; Garrard, P.; Buscema, M.; Dauwels, J.; Soekadar, S.R.; Mueller, S.; Linnemann, C.; et al. Innovative diagnostic tools for early detection of Alzheimer's disease. *Alzheimer's Dement.* **2015**, *11*, 561–578. [CrossRef]
15. Yim, D.; Yeo, T.Y.; Park, M.H. Mild cognitive impairment, dementia, and cognitive dysfunction screening using machine learning. *J. Int. Med. Res.* **2020**, *48*, 7. [CrossRef]
16. Schmid, N.S.; Taylor, K.I.; Foldi, N.S.; Berres, M.; Monsch, A.U. Neuropsychological signs of Alzheimer's disease 8 years prior to diagnosis. *J. Alzheimer's Dis.* **2013**, *34*, 537–546. [CrossRef]
17. Paúl, C.; Sousa, S.; Santos, P.; O'Caoimh, R.; Molloy, W. Screening Neurocognitive Disorders in Primary Care Services: The Quick Mild Cognitive Impairment Approach. *Innov. Aging* **2020**, *4*, 158. [CrossRef]
18. Murty, D.V.P.S.; Manikandan, K.; Kumar, W.S.; Ramesh, R.G.; Purokayastha, S.; Nagendra, B.; Ml, A.; Balakrishnan, A.; Javali, M.; Rao, N.P.; et al. Stimulus-induced gamma rhythms are weaker in human elderly with mild cognitive impairment and Alzheimer's disease. *eLife* **2021**, *10*, e61666. [CrossRef]
19. Oyama, A.; Takeda, S.; Ito, Y.; Nakajima, T.; Takami, Y.; Takeya, Y.; Yamamoto, K.; Sugimoto, K.; Shimizu, H.; Shimamura, M.; et al. Novel Method for Rapid Assessment of Cognitive Impairment Using High-Performance Eye-Tracking Technology. *Sci. Rep.* **2019**, *9*, 12932. [CrossRef]
20. Nie, J.; Qiu, Q.; Phillips, M.; Sun, L.; Yan, F.; Lin, X.; Xiao, S.; Li, X. Early Diagnosis of Mild Cognitive Impairment Based on Eye Movement Parameters in an Aging Chinese Population. *Front. Aging Neurosci.* **2020**, *12*, 221. [CrossRef]
21. Choi, J.; Lim, E.; Park, M.G.; Cha, W. Assessing the Retest Reliability of Prefrontal EEG Markers of Brain Rhythm Slowing in the Eyes-Closed Resting State. *Clin. EEG Neurosci.* **2020**, *51*, 348–356. [CrossRef]
22. Liu, Z.; Yang, Z.; Gu, Y.; Liu, H.; Wang, P. The effectiveness of eye tracking in the diagnosis of cognitive disorders: A systematic review and meta-analysis. *PLoS ONE* **2021**, *16*, e0254059. [CrossRef]
23. Jiang, J.; Yan, Z.; Sheng, C.; Wang, M.; Guan, Q.; Yu, Z.; Han, Y.; Jiang, J. A Novel Detection Tool for Mild Cognitive Impairment Patients Based on Eye Movement and Electroencephalogram. *J. Alzheimer's Dis.* **2019**, *72*, 389–399. [CrossRef]
24. Lv, S.; Wang, X.; Cui, Y.; Jin, J.; Sun, Y.L.; Tang, Y.; Bai, Y.; Wang, Y.; Zhou, L. Application of attention network test and demographic information to detect mild cognitive impairment via combining feature selection with support vector machine. *Comput. Methods Programs Biomed.* **2010**, *97*, 11–18. [CrossRef]
25. Lin, M.; Gong, P.; Yang, T.; Ye, J.; Albin, R.L.; Dodge, H.H.; Disorders, A. Big Data Analytical Approaches to the NACC Dataset: Aiding Preclinical Trial Enrichment. *Alzheimer Dis. Assoc. Disord.* **2018**, *32*, 18–27. [CrossRef]
26. Abásolo, D.E.; Hornero, R.; Espino, P.; Poza, J.; Sánchez, C.I.; Rosa, R. Analysis of regularity in the EEG background activity of Alzheimer's disease patients with Approximate Entropy. *Clin. Neurophysiol.* **2005**, *116*, 1826–1834. [CrossRef]
27. Costa, M.; Goldberger, A.L.; Peng, C.-K. Multiscale entropy analysis of complex physiologic time series. *Phys. Rev. Lett.* **2002**, *89*, 068102. [CrossRef]
28. Lempel, A.; Ziv, J. On the Complexity of Finite Sequences. *IEEE Trans. Inf. Theory* **1976**, *22*, 75–81. [CrossRef]
29. Peng, H.; Long, F.; Ding, C.; Intelligence, M. Feature selection based on mutual information criteria of max-dependency, max-relevance, and min-redundancy. *IEEE Trans. Pattern Anal. Mach. Intell.* **2005**, *27*, 1226–1238. [CrossRef]
30. Bondi, M.W.; Edmonds, E.C.; Jak, A.J.; Clark, L.; Delano-Wood, L.; McDonald, C.R.; Nation, D.A.; Libon, D.J.; Au, R.; Galasko, D.R.; et al. Neuropsychological criteria for mild cognitive impairment improves diagnostic precision, biomarker associations, and progression rates. *J. Alzheimer's Dis.* **2014**, *42*, 275–289. [CrossRef]

31. Albert, M.S.; DeKosky, S.T.; Dickson, D.W.; Dubois, B.; Feldman, H.H.; Fox, N.C.; Gamst, A.C.; Holtzman, D.M.; Jagust, W.J.; Petersen, R.C.; et al. The Diagnosis of Mild Cognitive Impairment due to Alzheimer's Disease: Recommendations from the National Institute on Aging-Alzheimer's Association Workgroups on Diagnostic Guidelines for Alzheimer's Disease. *Focus* **2011**, *11*, 96–106. [CrossRef]
32. Petersen, R.C. Mild cognitive impairment as a diagnostic entity. *Psychology* **2011**, *11*, 96–106. [CrossRef]
33. Siuly, S.; Alçin, Ö.F.; Kabir, E.; Şengür, A.; Wang, H.; Zhang, Y.; Whittaker, F.; Engineering, R. A New Framework for Automatic Detection of Patients With Mild Cognitive Impairment Using Resting-State EEG Signals. *IEEE Trans. Neural Syst. Rehabil. Eng.* **2020**, *28*, 1966–1976. [CrossRef]
34. Lagun, D.; Manzanares, C.; Zola, S.; Buffalo, E.; Agichtein, E. Detecting cognitive impairment by eye movement analysis using automatic classification algorithms. *J. Neurosci. Methods* **2011**, *201*, 196–203. [CrossRef]
35. Wang, J.; Wang, Z.; Liu, N.; Liu, C.; Mao, C.; Dong, L.-L.; Li, J.; Huang, X.; Lei, D.; Chu, S.; et al. Random Forest Model in the Diagnosis of Dementia Patients with Normal Mini-Mental State Examination Scores. *J. Pers. Med.* **2022**, *12*, 37. [CrossRef]

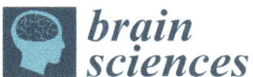

Article

A Novel Deep Learning Radiomics Model to Discriminate AD, MCI and NC: An Exploratory Study Based on Tau PET Scans from ADNI [†]

Yan Zhao [1,2,3,4,‡], Jieming Zhang [5,‡], Yue Chen [1,2,3,4,*] and Jiehui Jiang [1,6,*]

1. Nuclear Medicine and Molecular Imaging Key Laboratory of Sichuan Province, Luzhou 646000, China
2. Department of Nuclear Medicine, Affiliated Hospital of Southwest Medical University, Luzhou 646000, China
3. Institute of Nuclear Medicine, Southwest Medical University, Luzhou 646000, China
4. School of Pharmacy, Southwest Medical University, Luzhou 646000, China
5. School of Communication and Information Engineering, Shanghai University, Shanghai 200444, China
6. Institute of Biomedical Engineering, School of Life Science, Shanghai University, Shanghai 200444, China
* Correspondence: chenyue5523@126.com (Y.C.); jiangjiehui@shu.edu.cn (J.J.); Tel.: +86-137-009-898-31 (Y.C.); +86-139-189-209-26 (J.J.)
† For the Alzheimer's Disease Neuroimaging Initiative.
‡ The two authors contribute equally to this work.

Abstract: Objective: We explored a novel model based on deep learning radiomics (DLR) to differentiate Alzheimer's disease (AD) patients, mild cognitive impairment (MCI) patients and normal control (NC) subjects. This model was validated in an exploratory study using tau positron emission tomography (tau-PET) scans. Methods: In this study, we selected tau-PET scans from the Alzheimer's Disease Neuroimaging Initiative database (ADNI), which included a total of 211 NC, 197 MCI, and 117 AD subjects. The dataset was divided into one training/validation group and one separate external group for testing. The proposed DLR model contained the following three steps: (1) pre-training of candidate deep learning models; (2) extraction and selection of DLR features; (3) classification based on support vector machine (SVM). In the comparative experiments, we compared the DLR model with three traditional models, including the SUVR model, traditional radiomics model, and a clinical model. Ten-fold cross-validation was carried out 200 times in the experiments. Results: Compared with other models, the DLR model achieved the best classification performance, with an accuracy of 90.76% ± 2.15% in NC vs. MCI, 88.43% ± 2.32% in MCI vs. AD, and 99.92% ± 0.51% in NC vs. AD. Conclusions: Our proposed DLR model had the potential clinical value to discriminate AD, MCI and NC.

Keywords: Alzheimer's disease; mild cognitive impairment; tau positron emission tomography; deep learning radiomics

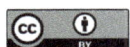

1. Introduction

Alzheimer's disease (AD) is the most prevalent cause of dementia and the most significant disease threatening the health of the elderly [1]. In the early stages of AD, patients often exhibit mild cognitive damage, i.e., mild memory loss mild executive function decrements (e.g., amyloid and tau pathological mechanism), and visuospatial impairment [2,3]. Mild cognitive impairment (MCI) is an intermediate step between normal aging and dementia [4], where patients start to appear memory impairment or other cognitive abnormalities, but have not reached the severity of dementia. Mild cognitive impairment subjects are at high-risk step for dementia [5]. Therefore, it is important to discriminate AD, MCI and normal control (NC) individuals [6,7].

tau positron emission tomography (tau-PET) imaging technology has become increasingly popular for the clinical diagnosis of AD and MCI [8–10]. The degree of brain tau accumulation, as an objective biomarker, is strongly correlated with the severity of AD.

Johnson et al. found that abnormally high cortical tau binding in the inferior temporal gyrus was associated with clinical impairment [11]. Zhao et al. found that typical deposits of tau appeared in the amygdala, entorhinal cortex, fusiform and parahippocampus in AD brains [12]. La Joie et al. included 28 AD patients and 25 patients with a non-AD clinical neurodegenerative diagnosis and found that tau-PET standard uptake value (SUVR) in the whole brain showed excellent discrimination power (area under curve (AUC) = 0.92–0.94) for diagnosing AD and MCI [13]. Sun et al. proposed a random forest diagnostic model for the classification of NC, MCI and AD and achieved an accuracy of 81.6% [14]. However, existing diagnosis models still have shortcomings, such as the need to manually extract features from the region of interest (ROI) and to encode the extracted features, which often requires tedious processes. Thus, an alternative approach is needed.

Deep learning radiomics (DLR) methods may be the alternative approach. DLR techniques are able to learn high-dimensional features from medical images autonomously and overcome shortcomings such as the cumbersome manual coding in traditional methods [15,16]. In recent years, DLR models have been used in AD studies [17,18]. For instance, Basaia et al. used a deep neural network to classify AD and MCI based on cross-sectional structural resonance imaging (MRI) images. The classification accuracy between AD and NC was 98.2%, and the accuracy of progression from MCI to AD was 74.9% [19]. Lee et al. employed a DLR model for AD classification based on MRI images and achieved an accuracy of 95.35% [20]. Pan et al. proposed a novel convolutional neural network (CNN) architecture called a multi-view separable pyramid network (MiSePyNet) and achieved a classification accuracy of 83.05% in predicting the progression from MCI to AD [21]. Lu et al. used multiscale neural networks to identify subjects with pre-symptomatic AD and achieved an accuracy of 82.51% based on 18F-fluorodeoxyglucose positron emission tomography (FDG-PET) images [22]. The above results showed the feasibility of DLR models for diagnosing AD and MCI. However, whether DLR models could be used to analyze tau-PET images is still unknown. Therefore, in this study, we assumed that the DLR technique was also feasible for application to tau-PET images and would be useful for the diagnosis of AD and MCI. To test the above hypothesis, we employed a novel DLR model and validated it in an exploratory study.

2. Methods and Materials

Figure 1 shows the whole experimental process of this study, which includes the following six steps: (1) subject enrollment; (2) tau-PET image preprocessing, including registration, smoothing, and numerical normalization; (3) deep learning (DL) model pre-training. During this session, several classical CNN models were selected and compared, and the best one was finally selected for the next step; (4) extraction of DLR features; (5) classification; (6) comparative experiments.

2.1. Subjects

The data used in this study were obtained from the ADNI cohort, which was jointly funded by the National Institutes of Health and the National Institute on Aging in 2004. ADNI is currently the definitive data center for AD-related disease research. In order to obtain the pathogenesis of AD and find treatments, ADNI aims to study the pathogenesis of AD and discover clinical, imaging, genetic and biochemical biomarkers that can be used for the early detection of AD by collecting and organizing longitudinal data from AD patients; the database currently has more than 2000 neuroimaging data. Specific information is available on ADNI's official website: http://adni.loni.usc.edu/about/, accessed on 12 November 2021.

In this study, a total of 211 NC subjects and 197 MCI and 117 AD patients were collected. All acquired subjects had both T1-weighted MRI images and tau-PET images. Of these, 189 NC subjects and 173 MCI and 101 AD patients were used to train and validate the DLR model. A separate 20 NC subjects and 18 MCI and 12 AD patients were used as an independent external test group. The remaining 2 NC subjects and 6 MCI and 4 AD patients were not included in the training or testing groups because images were found to be mutilated during pre-processing inspections. Demographic information (including gender, age and education) and T1-weighted MRI and tau-PET (AV 1451) images were collected for all participants. All subjects were also screened with the following neuropsychological examinations: the Clinical Dementia Rating-Sum of Boxes (CDR-SB), the MMSE, the MoCA-B, the 11-item and 13-item AD assessment cognitive scale (Alzheimer's disease assessment scale-cognitive, ADAS) and the ADAS delayed word recall (ADASQ4) subscale. Figure 2 shows the flow chart of the data inclusion/exclusion criteria.

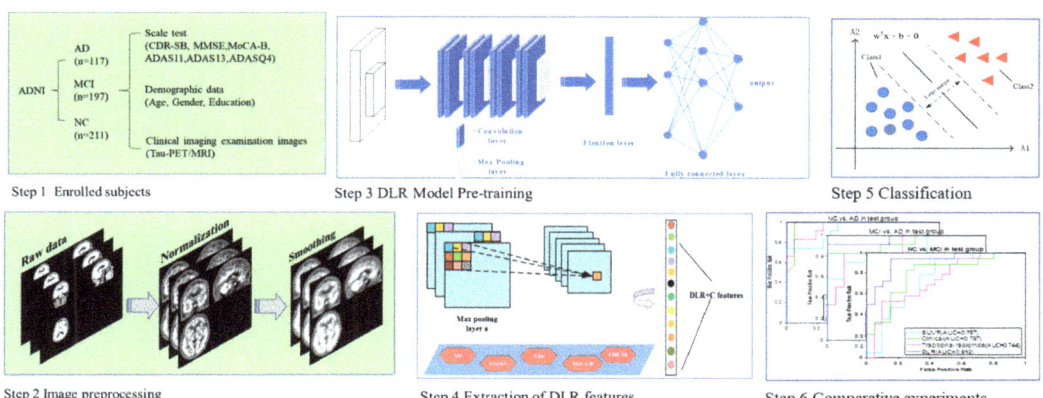

Figure 1. The whole experimental process in this study.

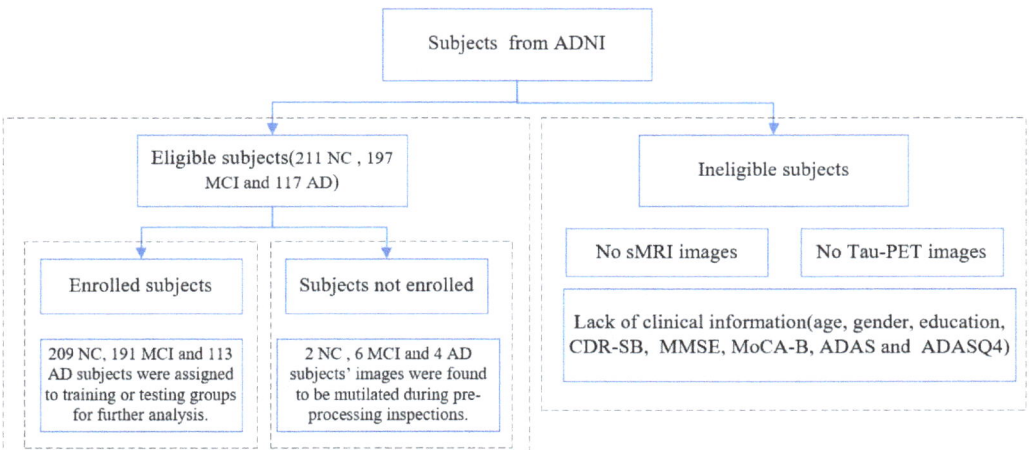

Figure 2. The flow chart of the data inclusion/exclusion criteria.

The inclusion criteria of MCI were according to the criteria proposed by Jak and Bondi in 2014 [5]: (1) Scores obtained in at least one cognitive domain (memory, language or speed, executive function) were below the standard deviation of the age/education corrected normative mean; (2) scores in each of the three cognitive domains of memory, language and speed/executive function were found to be impaired; (3) Scores on the Functional Activities Questionnaire (FAQ) ≥ 9. The diagnosis of AD was primarily based on guidelines provided by the National Institute on Aging (NIA) and the Alzheimer's Association (AA) working group. The ADNI institutional review board reviewed and approved the ADNI data collection protocol [7].

2.2. Images Acquisition and Preprocessing

The image acquisition process is described on the ADNI website at http://adni.loni.usc.edu/about/, accessed on 1 June 2021. All tau-PET images were preprocessed using SPM12 software (https://www.fil.ion.ucl.auk/spm/software/spm12/, accessed on 20 September 2021.) implemented in MATLAB 2019b. The preprocessing steps were as follows.

First, the DICOM images were uniformly converted to NIFTI format (.nii) using an image conversion tool for subsequent processing. The converted images were 3D image data with spatial structure information of the brain and retained the characteristic information between tissue structures. Second, since subjects might have some head tilt problems during tau-PET image acquisition, the original correction function in SPM12 was used in this experiment reduce external differences. Furthermore, the T1 MRI images were used to align the tau-PET images so that the corresponding points at spatially uniform locations in the two types of images corresponded to each other. Smoothing and numerical normalization were performed in the next step. After completing the above processing, the images were smoothed to suppress the noise, and the numerical normalization could eliminate the differences between different instruments and reduce the number of subsequent calculations. In this experiment, the images were normalized according to the tau-PET precipitated area in the cerebellar cortex region. After the above processing, 3D image data with a size of $91 \times 109 \times 91$ voxels in the standard space were obtained. To speed up the training time of the DLR models, all images were further normalized to -1 to 1 interval. In the unidirectional slicing condition, the 3D images were axially sliced into 91 single-channel images of size of 91×109 voxels, and the slices were filled and resampled to 224×224 voxels using linear interpolation due to the need to retain as much information as possible and to satisfy the model input conditions.

2.3. The Proposed DLR Model

The proposed DLR model is depicted in Figure 3. The model consists of the following steps: (1) DLR model pre-training. Five classical CNN networks were used for model pre-training. After comparison, we aimed to select the model with the best classification performance; (2) DLR feature extraction and fusion. Based on the pre-trained model, DLR features were extracted before the final maximum pooling layer and combined with clinical features; (3) classifiers: based on the features extracted above, support vector machine (SVM) was employed as the final classifier to obtain the classification results. The details of the model will be illustrated in the next sections.

2.3.1. DLR Model Pre-Training

In recent years, CNN models have been increasingly applied to medical imaging data and shown great potential in the classification tasks. In this study, we pre-trained five common CNN models, including AlexNet, ZF-Net, ResNet18, ResNet34, and InceptionV3 models.

(1) AlexNet demonstrates the excellent performance of deep CNN models. ReLU is used as the activation function for its network structure, which employs interleaved pooling in CNN models [23].
(2) ZF-Net is an improved CNN model based on AlexNet. Deconvolution is used to analyze feature behavior and then to improve classification performance [24].
(3) The Inception models have more complex network structures and unique network characteristics in comparison with AlexNet and ZF-Net. The Inception structure is designed to use multiple convolutional or pooling operations to form a network module. Inception V3, as the classic version of the Inception series, uses convolutional decomposition and regularization to enhance the classification performance [25].

(4) The ResNet framework introduces the residual network structure to solve the gradient disappearance or gradient explosion problem [26]. Different ResNet models, such as ResNet18, ResNet34, ResNet50 and ResNet101, are depending on the number of hidden layers. Figure 4 shows the structures of ResNet18 and ResNet34.

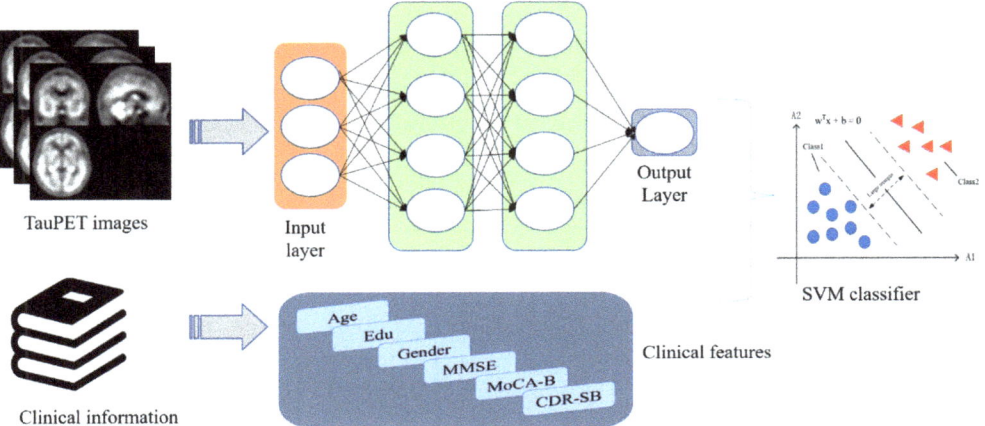

Figure 3. The framework of the proposed DLR model.

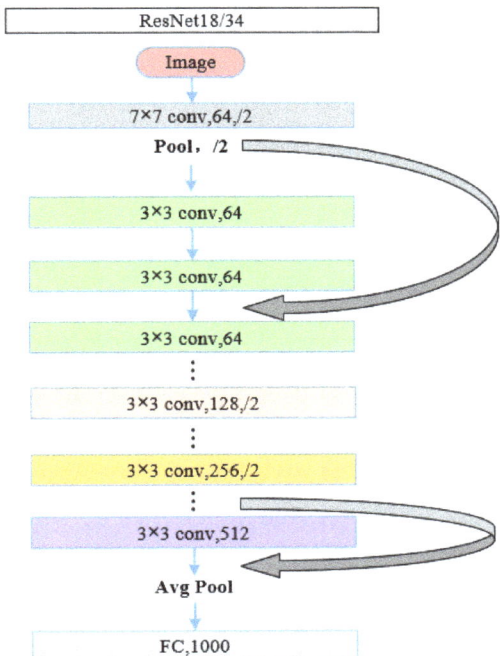

Figure 4. The fundamental structure of ResNet18 and ResNet34. "7 × 7" and "3 × 3" indicate the size of the convolution kernel, "conv" indicates convolution, "Avg Pool" indicates average pooling, and "FC" indicates fully connected layer. "64", "128", "128", "256" and "512" represent the numbers of channels, and "/2" means stride of 2.

The whole model pre-training process was divided into two parts: forward propagation and backward propagation. Before building the model, all tau-PET images were sliced and tiled into two-dimensional images and adjusted to 224 × 224 pixels. Then, all data were labeled using unique thermal coding. In the model pre-training step, all data were passed into the network and then converged using the stochastic gradient descent (SGD) algorithm and back propagated to update the model parameters. The final output of the model pre-training process was used as the classification result.

In the model pre-training step, we set the learning rate to 1×10^{-2} and updated the model parameters using an SGD optimizer with a batch size of 8. The number of training iterations was set to 100. In addition, we performed data enhancement in the training/validation group by flipping the images horizontally and adding Gaussian noise to the input images to prevent the overfitting problem. The above experiments were performed on GPU (graphics processing unit, RTX3090 accelerated by PyCharm 3.6 (JetBrains from the Czech Republic, website: https://www.jetbrains.com/pycharm/, accessed on 17 February 2022)).

2.3.2. DLR Feature Extraction and Fusion

In contrast to traditional methods relying on manually ROI segmentation, DLR methods can automatically leverage tau-PET images to obtain high-dimensional DLR features through supervised learning. After obtaining the best DL pre-trained model, we replaced the final maximum pooling layer and fully connected layer with the SVM as the final classifier. We extracted features from the last convolutional layer of each convolutional network. These features were treated as DLR features. Then, the clinical information (gender, age, education, CDR-SB, MoCA-B, MMSE, etc.) and the DLR features were combined as the input for the SVM classifier.

2.3.3. Classifier

SVM was used as the classifier in this study. SVM is essentially a linear classifier that maximizes intervals in feature space and is a binary classification model that has been widely used with statistical and regression analysis species [27]. We used a linear kernel as the kernel function.

2.4. Comparative Experiments

To demonstrate the superiority of the proposed DLR model, we compared the DLR model with three existing models, including: (1) The clinical model. This model includes demographic information and neuropsychological cognitive assessment tests as features for classification; (2) the standard uptake value ratio (SUVR) model. We calculated SUVR values of 10 tau-PET Meta ROIs as features for classification. The ten ROIs included inferior temporal lobe, lingual gyrus, middle temporal lobe, occipital lobe, parietal lobe, hippocampus, parahippocampus, posterior cingu late gyrus, precuneus and fusiform [28]; (3) the radiomics model. The radiomics features of the above 10 tau-PET Meta ROIs were extracted as features for classification. In this experiment, we used the Radiomics Toolkit (https://github.com/mvallieres/radiomics, accessed on 17 February 2022) to extract radiomics features. The feature extraction steps included wavelet band-pass filtering, isotropic resampling, Lloyd–Max quantization, feature computation, and so on [29,30]. In the comparison experiments, each model was with 10-fold cross-validation 200 times.

2.5. Statistical Analysis

In this study, chi-square tests and nonparametric rank sum tests were introduced to compare differences in demographic characteristics between the training/validation group and the test group. We used SPSS version 25.0 software (SPSS Inc., Chicago, IL, USA) for all statistical analyses. Statistical results with p values < 0.05 were considered significantly different.

3. Results

3.1. Subject Demographics

Table 1 shows the demographic results. There were differences in MoCA-B ($p = 0.042$) and age ($p = 0.03$) in the NC group; ADAS11 ($p = 0.020$), ADAS13 ($p = 0.034$) and ADASQ4 ($p = 0.044$) in the MCI group and no significant differences in the AD group.

Table 1. Demographic information in this study.

	NC Groups		MCI Groups		AD Groups	
	NC1 (Train)	NC2 (Test)	MCI1 (Train)	MCI2 (Test)	AD1 (Train)	AD2 (Test)
Gender (M/F)	69/121	10/11	95/83	13/6	62/43	5/7
Age (year)	73.17 ± 7.64	76.76 ± 6.85 [a]	73.88 ± 7.46	70.93 ± 8.21	75.39 ± 7.94	76.76 ± 9.38
Education	16.66 ± 2.34	17.10 ± 2.04	16.39 ± 2.56	16.05 ± 2.37	15.49 ± 2.59	15.33 ± 2.61
MMSE	29.11 ± 1.23	29.14 ± 1.06	27.78 ± 2.21	27.37 ± 2.31	21.36 ± 4.98	21.58 ± 3.55
MoCA-B	26.36 ± 2.55	25.00 ± 2.73 [a]	23.24 ± 3.54	23.68 ± 3.16	16.15 ± 5.03	16.20 ± 4.64
CDR-SB	0.06 ± 0.23	0.10 ± 0.20	1.45 ± 1.03	2.37 ± 1.88	5.92 ± 3.32	5.13 ± 2.22
ADAS11	8.69 ± 2.57	8.93 ± 1.86	12.59 ± 4.11	14.25 ± 3.08 [a]	22.10 ± 7.29	25.03 ± 5.98
ADAS13	12.46 ± 4.12	13.25 ± 2.99	19.01 ± 6.11	21.51 ± 5.10 [a]	32.57 ± 8.64	36.11 ± 7.20
ADASQ4	2.51 ± 1.72	3.25 ± 2.00	4.77 ± 2.26	5.89 ± 2.35 [a]	8.06 ± 1.32	8.25 ± 1.76

[a] indicated that the p value was less than 0.05 in comparison results between the training/validation and test groups under the same label.

All data are expressed as mean ± standard deviation. MMSE, Mini-mental State Examination; MoCA-B, Montreal cognitive assessment-basic; CDR-SB, clinical dementia rating sum of boxes; ADAS11 and ADAS13, the 11-item and 13-item AD assessment scale cognitive; ADASQ4, the ADAS delayed word recall subscale.

For age, education, MMSE, MoCA-B, CDR-SB, ADAS11, ADAS13 and ADASQ4, a nonparametric rank sum test was performed to compare differences in demographic and clinical characteristics between the training/validation and test groups under each label, i.e., NC, MCI and AD; gender was tested by chi-square between the two groups under each label.

3.2. Pre-Training Results of Candidate DL Models

Tables 2–4 present the classification performance of the five candidate DL models. The performance evaluation metrics include accuracy, sensitivity and specificity. ResNet18 had the highest classification performance in NC vs. MCI, while ResNet34 had the highest classification performance in MCI vs. AD and NC vs. AD. Therefore, ResNet34 was selected to extract the corresponding DLR features.

Table 2. Classification performance in NC vs. MCI.

Model	Accuracy (%)	Sensitivity (%)	Specificity (%)
Training/Validation Groups			
AlexNet	94.26 ± 2.60	93.80 ± 2.92	94.70 ± 4.34
ZF-Net	94.28 ± 3.99	94.97 ± 3.64	93.66 ± 7.46
ResNet18	95.78 ± 2.50	94.99 ± 4.70	96.51 ± 2.98
ResNet34	95.32 ± 2.62	94.06 ± 3.74	96.49 ± 4.55
InceptionV3	93.82 ± 3.94	93.02 ± 4.93	94.54 ± 6.39
Test Group			
AlexNet	81.25 ± 3.06	7947 ± 2.86	82.86 ± 3.83
ZF-Net	83.14 ± 3.24	78.37 ± 3.89	86.67 ± 5.95
ResNet18	**87.25 ± 2.21**	**87.37 ± 2.24**	**87.14 ± 2.32**
ResNet34	87.00 ± 2.14	85.79 ± 2.12	88.10 ± 2.52
InceptionV3	80.50 ± 3.58	77.89 ± 4.24	82.86 ± 5.79

The bold means this model performed best among others.

Table 3. Classification performance in MCI vs. AD.

Model	Accuracy (%)	Sensitivity (%)	Specificity (%)
Training/Validation Groups			
AlexNet	93.18 ± 4.36	89.33 ± 10.55	95.41 ± 3.59
ZF-Net	93.55 ± 5.19	91.37 ± 7.20	94.77 ± 5.16
ResNet18	93.72 ± 3.40	90.47 ± 8.16	95.63 ± 4.22
ResNet34	95.28 ± 2.50	94.76 ± 4.96	95.59 ± 3.03
InceptionV3	97.45 ± 2.78	95.26 ± 6.77	98.75 ± 2.64
Test Group			
AlexNet	79.68 ± 5.12	64.17 ± 7.32	89.47 ± 4.81
ZF-Net	79.68 ± 2.40	62.50 ± 3.78	90.52 ± 2.34
ResNet18	82.26 ± 1.78	73.33 ± 2.72	87.89 ± 2.14
ResNet34	**82.26 ± 1.54**	**77.50 ± 2.48**	**85.26 ± 2.12**
InceptionV3	79.68 ± 2.14	74.17 ± 3.32	83.16 ± 3.48

The bold means this model performed best among others.

Table 4. Classification performance in NC vs. AD.

Model	Accuracy (%)	Sensitivity (%)	Specificity (%)
Training/Validation Groups			
AlexNet	97.36 ± 2.98	95.67 ± 7.25	98.27 ± 2.44
ZF-Net	98.30 ± 2.42	97.89 ± 5.09	98.53 ± 2.08
ResNet18	97.17 ± 2.05	96.87 ± 4.42	97.32 ± 2.60
ResNet34	98.10 ± 1.81	96.14 ± 5.87	99.14 ± 1.38
InceptionV3	94.37 ± 3.53	91.29 ± 8.66	96.16 ± 3.13
Test Group			
AlexNet	94.24 ± 0.96	84.17 ± 2.63	100.0 ± 0.00
ZF-Net	93.64 ± 2.65	82.57 ± 7.34	100.0 ± 0.00
ResNet18	96.97 ± 2.91	91.70 ± 3.50	100.0 ± 0.00
ResNet34	**96.97 ± 2.16**	**91.70 ± 2.83**	**100.0 ± 0.00**
InceptionV3	95.08 ± 3.14	89.58 ± 5.30	98.21 ± 0.96

The bold means this model performed best among others.

3.3. Comparative Experiments

3.3.1. NC vs. MCI

Table 5 shows the classification results of the four models in NC vs. MCI. The DLR model performed the best classification performance, with an accuracy of 90.76% ± 2.15%, sensitivity of 94.17% ± 1.81% and specificity of 87.74% ± 2.54% in the test group. The remaining three models performed obviously lower than the DLR model with accuracy of 75.68% ± 2.63%, 72.02% ± 4.12% and 81.61% ± 3.23%; sensitivity of 62.32% ± 4.52%, 68.95% ± 9.22% and 83.11% ± 3.14%; and specificity of 86.67% ± 2.92%, 74.76% ± 7.11% and 80.31% ± 6.38%.

Figure 5 provides the ROC curves of the four models. The AUC (mean ± SD) for the DLR model reached 0.922 ± 0.021 and achieved the best performance among these models.

3.3.2. MCI vs. AD

Table 6 shows the classification performance of the four models in MCI vs. AD. The DLR model showed accuracy of 88.43% ± 2.32%, sensitivity of 91.25% ± 2.05% and specificity of 86.56% ± 2.86% in the test group. The remaining three models performed obviously lower than the DLR model with accuracy of 78.33% ± 4.27%, 79.68% ± 5.72% and 77.16% ± 2.95%; sensitivity of 62.67% ± 9.12%, 65.63% ± 10.97% and 88.17% ± 9.25%; and specificity of 86.67% ± 2.92%, 88.95% ± 2.99% and 68.91% ± 7.64%, respectively.

Table 5. The classification performance in NC vs. MCI.

Model	Accuracy (%)	Sensitivity (%)	Specificity (%)
Training/Validation Groups			
SUVR model	69.36 ± 7.94	63.53 ± 12.03	74.73 ± 10.74
Traditional radiomics model	69.05 ± 7.22	63.34 ± 13.34	74.28 ± 7.07
Clinical model	74.84 ± 8.48	80.13 ± 14.16	71.58 ± 12.05
DLR model	**98.46 ± 1.71**	**98.47 ± 1.66**	**98.44 ± 1.76**
Test Group			
SUVR model	75.68 ± 2.63	62.32 ± 4.52	86.67 ± 2.92
Traditional radiomics model	72.02 ± 4.12	68.95 ± 9.22	74.76 ± 7.11
Clinical model	81.61 ± 3.23	83.11 ± 3.14	80.31 ± 6.38
DLR model	**90.76 ± 2.15**	**94.74 ± 1.81**	**87.74 ± 2.54**

The bold means this model performed best among others.

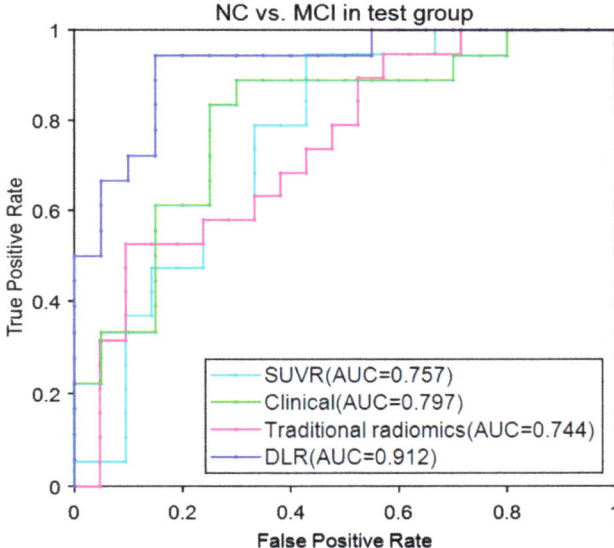

Figure 5. ROC curves for the four models in NC vs. MCI.

Table 6. The classification performance in MCI vs. AD.

Model	Accuracy (%)	Sensitivity (%)	Specificity (%)
Training/Validation Groups			
SUVR model	74.41 ± 8.15	55.39 ± 15.64	86.06 ± 8.88
Traditional radiomics model	70.20 ± 7.83	57.79 ± 13.64	81.58 ± 9.83
Clinical model	90.84 ± 4.95	84.59 ± 11.04	94.45 ± 5.00
DLR model	**96.27 ± 1.16**	**94.90 ± 4.81**	**97.89 ± 2.11**
Test Group			
SUVR model	78.33 ± 4.27	62.67 ± 9.12	86.67 ± 2.92
Traditional radiomics model	79.68 ± 5.72	65.63 ± 10.97	88.95 ± 2.99
Clinical model	77.16 ± 2.95	88.17 ± 9.25	68.91 ± 7.64
DLR model	**88.43 ± 2.32**	**91.25 ± 2.05**	**86.56 ± 2.86**

The bold means this model performed best among others.

Figure 6 provided the ROC curves of these four models. The AUC (mean ± SD) for the DLR model reached 0.928 ± 0.024 and achieved the best performance among these models.

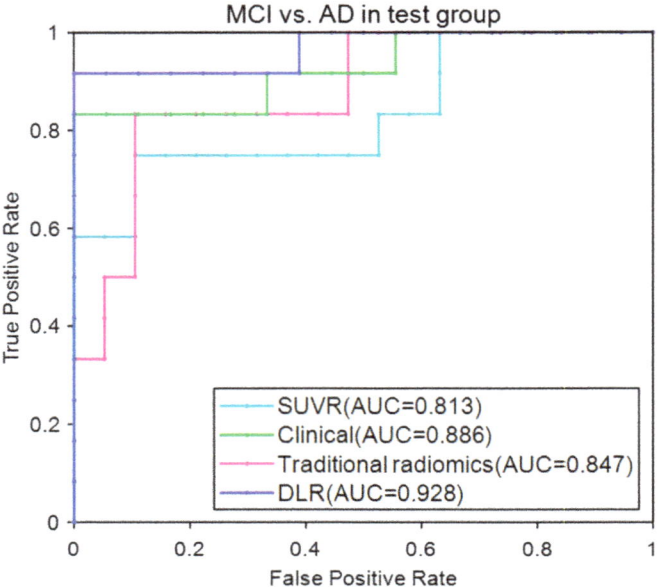

Figure 6. ROC curves for the four models in MCI vs. AD.

3.3.3. NC vs. AD

Table 7 shows the classification performance of the four models in MCI vs. AD. The DLR model showed an accuracy of 99.92% ± 0.51%, sensitivity of 99.78% ± 0.13%, and specificity of 99.99% ± 0.14% in the test group. The remaining three models performed obviously lower than the DLR model with accuracy of 90.66% ± 0.85%, 87.58% ± 3.63% and 96.98% ± 0.21%; sensitivity of 74.96% ± 0.59%, 74.17% ± 9.43% and 92.78% ± 3.13%; and specificity of 99.63% ± 1.33%, 95.24% ± 3.17% and 99.56% ± 2.17%.

Table 7. The classification performance in NC vs. AD.

Model	Accuracy (%)	Sensitivity (%)	Specificity (%)
Training/Validation Groups			
SUVR model	86.06 ± 6.18	73.43 ± 14.21	93.04 ± 6.06
Traditional radiomics model	78.65 ± 0.08	57.67 ± 16.64	87.06 ± 8.80
Clinical model	91.96 ± 5.44	99.06 ± 2.98	86.65 ± 8.04
DLR model	**99.31 ± 1.50**	**98.00 ± 4.43**	**100.0 ± 0.00**
Test Group			
SUVR model	90.66 ± 0.85	74.96 ± 0.59	99.63 ± 1.33
Traditional radiomics model	85.58 ± 3.63	74.17 ± 9.43	95.24 ± 3.17
Clinical model	96.98 ± 0.21	92.78 ± 3.13	99.56 ± 2.17
DLR model	**99.92 ± 0.51**	**99.78 ± 0. 13**	**99.99 ± 0.14**

The bold means this model performed best among others.

Figure 7 provided the ROC curves of these four models. The AUC (mean ± SD) for the DLR model reached 0.996 ± 0.002 and achieved the best performance among these models.

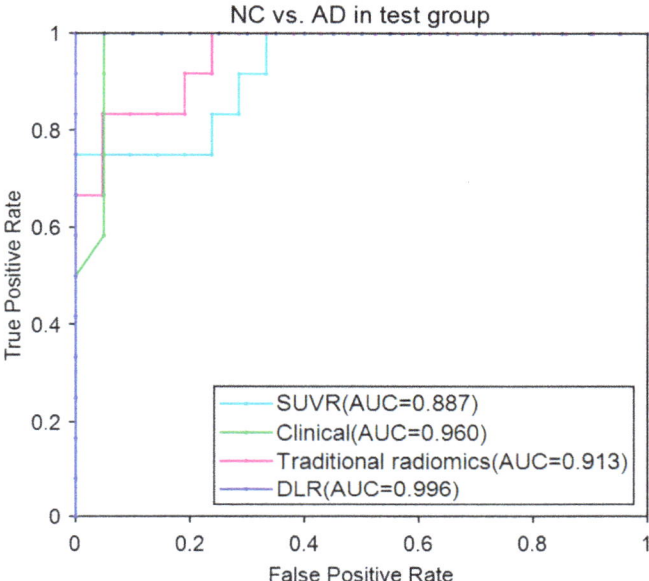

Figure 7. ROC curves for the four models in NC vs. AD.

4. Discussion

DLR has been becoming a hot topic nowadays. Because of its excellent performance in image recognition and processing, DLR models have been commonly used in computer-aided disease diagnostic fields such lesion detection, quantitative lesion diagnosis, treatment decision and prognosis expectation. In this study, we proposed a DLR model based on tau-PET images to distinguish NC, MCI and AD. In contrast with other traditional models, such as the SUVR model, the traditional radiomics model and the clinical model, the DLR model achieved the best classification results.

To date, many studies have focused on the classification among NC, MCI and AD using machine learning or DL models. For instance, Lange et al. performed a voxel-based statistical analysis using FDG-PET images and achieved an AUC of 0.728 in the classification of AD and NC [31]. Zhou et al. fused MRI and FDG-PET images and used radiomics analysis to achieve an accuracy of 0.733 in the classification of MCI and NC [32]. Shu et al. used radiomics features based on MRI images to classify MCI and AD and achieved an accuracy of 0.807 [33].

Compared with previous studies, our proposed DLR model achieved superior classification results (90.76% ± 2.15% in NC vs. MCI, 88.43% ± 2.32% in MCI vs. AD, and 99.92% ± 0.51% in NC vs. AD). The reasons may be as follows: (1) The DLR model is able to extract deeper image feature information from the pre-processed tau-PET images. As it does not require an additional ROI segmentation step, it decreases errors and biases caused by ROI segmentation; (2) the DLR model is subject to unavoidable external influences such as individual differences and different parameters of imaging acquisition. In our experiment, the DLR features and clinical information were combined together, so bias caused by individual heterogeneities may be eliminated.

Although the DLR model achieved good classification results, several limitations still exist. First, more supporting data are needed to verify the stability of our proposed DLR model. In this research, all data were obtained from the ADNI database. It is worth exploring whether our model works well with other databases. We only used the ADNI database, and the robustness of the results needs to be further verified. In the future, we plan to incorporate other ethnic group data to further verify the effectiveness of our model.

Second, we only adopted five classical deep convolutional networks to obtain the final DLR model. Although the ResNet models performed well in this classification experiment, there may be other more suitable models that can be applied. Moreover, we used whole-brain tau-PET images to train the model, and it remains to be explored whether extracting ROIs would yield better results. In addition to this, in this experiment, the 3D tau-PET images were segmented and sliced according to the axial direction. Whether better results can be obtained using 3D images and convolutional networks at the 3D level requires further validation and experiments. Finally, the model is trained on tau-PET images. Combining with other modalities, such as amyloid PET, MRI and FDG-PET images may improve the classification accuracy. In summary, the DLR model we proposed in this study provides a certain help with the clinical diagnosis and differentiation of NC, MCI and AD. Through this tau-Pet image-based DLR-assisted diagnosis of MCI, early intervention can be carried out for the MCI population, which can improve the cognitive function of patients, allow for early treatment and delay the conversion to dementia.

5. Conclusions

In this study, we developed a tau-PET-based DLR method for the subgroup diagnosis of NC, MCI and AD. This study shows that the proposed DLR method can improve the diagnostic performance of MCI and AD patients and provide the possibility of MCI-to-AD conversion prediction. In the future, the DLR method will propose practical applications for the computer-aided diagnosis of MCI and AD. We believe that more image modalities based on our proposed DLR method will be applied in the differential diagnosis of NC, MCI and AD.

Author Contributions: Y.Z. and J.Z. carried out the whole experiment together and and co-wrote the manuscript. During the experiment, Y.Z. conducted the data collecting and management. J.Z. focused on data analysis and programming the code to obtain the final results. During the writing phase, Y.Z. mainly focused on the Introduction and Discussion sections, and J.Z. focused on the Methods and Results sections. Y.C. and J.J. presented the idea and performed the conceptualization and supervision. All authors have read and agreed to the published version of the manuscript.

Funding: This study was supported by the Open Project Program of Nuclear Medicine and Molecular Imaging Key Laboratory of Sichuan Province (HYX21004).

Institutional Review Board Statement: The data for this article was collected from ADNI. The ADNI study was conducted according to Good Clinical Practice guidelines, the Declaration of Helsinki, US 21CFR Part 50—Protection of Human Subjects, and Part 56—Institutional Review Boards, and pursuant to state and federal HIPAA regulations. Each participating site obtained ethical approval from their Institutional Review Board before commencing subject enrolment.

Informed Consent Statement: Informed consent was obtained from all subjects involved in the study. The human data was acquired from the publicly available ADNI database which meet the ethics requirements.

Data Availability Statement: The subject data used in this study were obtained from the Alzheimer's Disease Neuroimaging Initiative (ADNI) database (adni.loni.usc.edu). Meanwhile, data supporting the findings of this study are available from the corresponding authors upon reasonable request.

Acknowledgments: Data sources and collection for this paper were supported by the Alzheimer's Disease Neuroimaging Initiative (ADNI; National Institutes of Health Grant U01 AG024904) and the DODADNI (Department of Defense, award number W81XWH-12–2-0012). ADNI is funded by the National Institute of Aging and the National Institute of Biomedical Imaging and Bioengineering and through generous contributions from the following: AbbVie, Alzheimer's Association; Alzheimer's Drug Discovery Foundation; Araclon Biotech; BioClinica Inc; Biogen; Bristol-Myers Squibb Company; CereSpir Inc.; Eisai Inc.; Elan Pharmaceuticals Inc.; Eli Lilly and Company; EuroImmun; F.Hoffmann-La Roche Ltd. and its affiliated company Genentech Inc; Fujirebio; GE Healthcare; IXICO Ltd.; Janssen Alzheimer Immunotherapy Research & Development, LLC.; Johnson & Johnson Pharmaceutical

Research & Development LLC.; Lumosity; Lundbeck; Merck & Co., Inc.; Meso Scale Diagnostics, LLC; NeuroRx Research; Neu-rotrack Technologies; Novartis Pharmaceuticals Corporation; Pfizer Inc; Piramal Imaging; Servier; Takeda Pharmaceutical Company; and Transition Therapeutics. The Canadian Institutes of Health Research is providing funds to support ADNI clinical sites in Canada.

Conflicts of Interest: The authors declare that this study was conducted without any commercial or financial relationship that could be considered a potential conflict of interest.

References

1. Alzheimer's Association. 2017 Alzheimer's disease facts and figures. *Alzheimers Dement.* **2017**, *13*, 325–373. [CrossRef]
2. Morris, J.C.; Storandt, M.; Miller, J.P.; McKeel, D.W.; Price, J.L.; Rubin, E.H.; Berg, L. Mild Cognitive Impairment Represents Early-Stage Alzheimer Disease. *Arch. Neurol.* **2001**, *58*, 397–405. [CrossRef]
3. Petersen, R.C. Mild cognitive impairment as a diagnostic entity. *J. Intern. Med.* **2004**, *256*, 183–194. [CrossRef]
4. Winblad, B.; Palmer, K.; Kivipelto, M.; Jelic, V.; Fratiglioni, L.; Wahlund, L.-O.; Nordberg, A.; Backman, L.J.; Albert, M.S.; Almkvist, O.; et al. Mild cognitive impairment—Beyond controversies, towards a consensus: Report of the International Working Group on Mild Cognitive Impairment. *J. Intern. Med.* **2004**, *256*, 240–246. [CrossRef] [PubMed]
5. Bondi, M.W.; Edmonds, E.C.; Jak, A.J.; Clark, L.R.; Delano-Wood, L.; McDonald, C.R.; Nation, D.A.; Libon, D.J.; Au, R.; Galasko, D.; et al. Neuropsychological Criteria for Mild Cognitive Impairment Improves Diagnostic Precision, Biomarker Associations, and Progression Rates. *J. Alzheimer's Dis.* **2014**, *42*, 275–289. [CrossRef]
6. Albert, M.S.; DeKosky, S.T.; Dickson, D.; Dubois, B.; Feldman, H.H.; Fox, N.C.; Gamst, A.; Holtzman, D.M.; Jagust, W.J.; Petersen, R.C.; et al. The diagnosis of mild cognitive impairment due to Alzheimer's disease: Recommendations from the National Institute on Aging-Alzheimer's Association workgroups on diagnostic guidelines for Alzheimer's disease. *Alzheimers Dement.* **2011**, *7*, 270–279. [CrossRef] [PubMed]
7. McKhann, G.M.; Knopman, D.S.; Chertkow, H.; Hyman, B.T.; Jack, C.R., Jr.; Kawas, C.H.; Klunk, W.E.; Koroshetz, W.J.; Manly, J.J.; Mayeux, R.; et al. The diagnosis of dementia due to Alzheimer's disease: Recommendations from the National Institute on Aging-Alzheimer's association workgroups on diagnostic guidelines for Alzheimer's disease. *Alzheimers Dement. J. Alzheimers Assoc.* **2011**, *7*, 263–269. [CrossRef]
8. Campese, N.; Palermo, G.; Del Gamba, C.; Beatino, M.F.; Galgani, A.; Belli, E.; Del Prete, E.; Della Vecchia, A.; Vergallo, A.; Siciliano, G.; et al. Progress regarding the context-of-use of tau as biomarker of Alzheimer's disease and other neurodegenerative diseases. *Expert Rev. Proteom.* **2021**, *18*, 27–48. [CrossRef]
9. Jack, C.R., Jr.; Bennett, D.A.; Blennow, K.; Carrillo, M.C.; Dunn, B.; Haeberlein, S.B.; Holtzman, D.M.; Jagust, W.; Jessen, F.; Karlawish, J.; et al. NIA-AA Research Framework: Toward a biological definition of Alzheimer's disease. *Alzheimer Dement.* **2018**, *14*, 535–562. [CrossRef]
10. Lloret, A.; Esteve, D.; Cervera-Ferri, A.; Lopez, B.; Nepomuceno, M.; Monllor, P. When Does Alzheimer's Disease Really Start? The Role of Biomarkers. *Int. J. Mol. Sci.* **2019**, *20*, 5536. [CrossRef]
11. Johnson, K.A.; Schultz, A.; Betensky, R.A.; Becker, J.A.; Sepulcre, J.; Rentz, D.M.; Mormino, E.C.; Chhatwal, J.; Amariglio, R.; Papp, K.; et al. Tau positron emission tomographic imaging in aging and early Alzheimer disease. *Ann. Neurol.* **2015**, *79*, 110–119. [CrossRef] [PubMed]
12. Zhao, Q.; Liu, M.; Ha, L.; Zhou, Y.; Initiative, A.D.N.; Weiner, M.W.; Aisen, P.; Petersen, R.; Jack, C.R.J.; Jagust, W.; et al. Quantitative 18F-AV1451 Brain Tau PET Imaging in Cognitively Normal Older Adults, Mild Cognitive Impairment, and Alzheimer's Disease Patients. *Front. Neurol.* **2019**, *10*, 486. [CrossRef] [PubMed]
13. La Joie, R.; Bejanin, A.; Fagan, A.M.; Ayakta, N.; Baker, S.L.; Bourakova, V.; Boxer, A.L.; Cha, J.; Karydas, A.; Jerome, G.; et al. Associations between [18F]AV1451 tau PET and CSF measures of tau pathology in a clinical sample. *Neurology* **2017**, *90*, e282–e290. [CrossRef] [PubMed]
14. Sun, H.; Wang, A.; Ai, Q.; Wang, Y. A New-Style Random Forest Diagnosis Model for Alzheimer's Disease. *J. Med. Imaging Health Inform.* **2020**, *10*, 705–709. [CrossRef]
15. Liu, Z.; Wang, S.; Dong, D.; Wei, J.; Fang, C.; Zhou, X.; Sun, K.; Li, L.; Li, B.; Wang, M.; et al. The Applications of Radiomics in Precision Diagnosis and Treatment of Oncology: Opportunities and Challenges. *Theranostics* **2019**, *9*, 1303–1322. [CrossRef] [PubMed]
16. Suzuki, K. Overview of deep learning in medical imaging. *Radiol. Phys. Technol.* **2017**, *10*, 257–273. [CrossRef] [PubMed]
17. Li, Y.; Wei, D.; Liu, X.; Fan, X.; Wang, K.; Li, S.; Zhang, Z.; Ma, K.; Qian, T.; Jiang, T.; et al. Molecular subtyping of diffuse gliomas using magnetic resonance imaging: Comparison and correlation between radiomics and deep learning. *Eur. Radiol.* **2021**, *32*, 747–758. [CrossRef]
18. Park, J.E.; Kickingereder, P.; Kim, H.S. Radiomics and Deep Learning from Research to Clinical Workflow: Neuro-Oncologic Imaging. *Korean J. Radiol.* **2020**, *21*, 1126. [CrossRef] [PubMed]
19. Basaia, S.; Agosta, F.; Wagner, L.; Canu, E.; Magnani, G.; Santangelo, R.; Filippi, M. Automated classification of Alzheimer's disease and mild cognitive impairment using a single MRI and deep neural networks. *NeuroImage Clin.* **2018**, *21*, 101645. [CrossRef] [PubMed]

20. Lee, B.; Ellahi, W.; Choi, J.Y. Using Deep CNN with Data Permutation Scheme for Classification of Alzheimer's Disease in Structural Magnetic Resonance Imaging (sMRI). *IEICE Trans. Inf. Syst.* **2019**, *E102D*, 1384–1395. [CrossRef]
21. Pan, X.; Phan, T.-L.; Adel, M.; Fossati, C.; Gaidon, T.; Wojak, J.; Guedj, E. Multi-View Separable Pyramid Network for AD Prediction at MCI Stage by ^{18}F-FDG Brain PET Imaging. *IEEE Trans. Med. Imaging* **2020**, *40*, 81–92. [CrossRef]
22. Lu, D.; Popuri, K.; Ding, G.W.; Balachandar, R.; Beg, M.F. Multiscale deep neural network based analysis of FDG-PET images for the early diagnosis of Alzheimer's disease. *Med. Image Anal.* **2018**, *46*, 26–34. [CrossRef] [PubMed]
23. Krizhevsky, A.; Sutskever, I.; Hinton, G.E. Imagenet classification with deep convolutional neural networks. *NIPS* **2012**, *60*, 84–90. [CrossRef]
24. Zeiler, M.; Fergus, R. *Visualizing and Understanding Convolutional Networks*; Fleet, D., Pajdla, T., Schiele, B., Tuytelaars, T., Eds.; Springer: Berlin/Heidelberg, Germany, 2014; Volume 8689, pp. 818–833.
25. Szegedy, C.; Vanhoucke, V.; Ioffe, S.; Shlens, J.; Wojna, Z. Rethinking the Inception Architecture for Computer Vision. In Proceedings of the IEEE Conference on Computer Vision and Pattern Recognition, Las Vegas, NV, USA, 27–30 June 2016; pp. 2818–2826.
26. He, K.; Zhang, X.; Ren, S.; Sun, J. Deep Residual Learning for Image Recognition. In Proceedings of the IEEE Conference on Computer Vision and Pattern Recognition, Las Vegas, NV, USA, 27–30 June 2016; pp. 770–778.
27. Amari, S.; Wu, S. Improving support vector machine classifiers by modifying kernel functions. *Neural Netw.* **1999**, *12*, 783–789. [CrossRef]
28. Chotipanich, C.; Nivorn, M.; Kunawudhi, A.; Promteangtrong, C.; Boonkawin, N.; Jantarato, A. Evaluation of Imaging Windows for Tau PET Imaging Using ^{18}F-PI2620 in Cognitively Normal Individuals, Mild Cognitive Impairment, and Alzheimer's Disease Patients. *Mol. Imaging* **2020**, *19*, 1–8. [CrossRef] [PubMed]
29. Gillies, R.J.; Kinahan, P.E.; Hricak, H. Radiomics: Images Are More than Pictures, They Are Data. *Radiology* **2016**, *278*, 563–577. [CrossRef]
30. Kumar, V.; Gu, Y.; Basu, S.; Berglund, A.; Eschrich, S.A.; Schabath, M.B.; Forster, K.; Aerts, H.J.W.L.; Dekker, A.; Fenstermacher, D.; et al. Radiomics: The process and the challenges. *Magn. Reson. Imaging* **2012**, *30*, 1234–1248. [CrossRef]
31. Lange, C.; Suppa, P.; Frings, L.; Brenner, W.; Spies, L.; Buchert, R. Optimization of Statistical Single Subject Analysis of Brain FDG PET for the Prognosis of Mild Cognitive Impairment-to-Alzheimer's Disease Conversion. *J. Alzheimer's Dis.* **2016**, *49*, 945–959. [CrossRef]
32. Zhou, H.; Jiang, J.; Lu, J.; Wang, M.; Zhang, H.; Zuo, C.; Initiative, A.D.N. Dual-Model Radiomic Biomarkers Predict Development of Mild Cognitive Impairment Progression to Alzheimer's Disease. *Front. Neurosci.* **2019**, *12*, 1045. [CrossRef]
33. Shu, Z.-Y.; Mao, D.-W.; Xu, Y.-Y.; Shao, Y.; Pang, P.-P.; Gong, X.-Y. Prediction of the progression from mild cognitive impairment to Alzheimer's disease using a radiomics-integrated model. *Ther. Adv. Neurol. Disord.* **2021**, *14*, 1–13. [CrossRef]

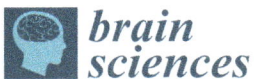

Article

In Vivo Tau Burden Is Associated with Abnormal Brain Functional Connectivity in Alzheimer's Disease: A ^{18}F-Florzolotau Study

Zizhao Ju [1,†], Zhuoyuan Li [2,†], Jiaying Lu [1], Fangyang Jiao [1], Huamei Lin [1], Weiqi Bao [1], Ming Li [1], Ping Wu [1], Yihui Guan [1], Qianhua Zhao [3], Huiwei Zhang [1,*], Jiehui Jiang [4,*] and Chuantao Zuo [1]

[1] PET Center and National Research Center for Aging and Medicine & National Center for Neurological Disorders, Huashan Hospital, Fudan University, Shanghai 200035, China
[2] School of Communication and Information Engineering, Shanghai University, Shanghai 200444, China
[3] Department of Neurology, Huashan Hospital, Fudan University, Shanghai 200040, China
[4] Institute of Biomedical Engineering, School of Life Science, Shanghai University, Shanghai 200444, China
* Correspondence: zhanghuiwei@fudan.edu.cn (H.Z.); jiangjiehui@shu.edu.cn (J.J.)
† These authors contributed equally to this work.

Abstract: Purpose: ^{18}F-Florzolotau is a novel second-generation tau radiotracer that shows higher binding affinity and selectivity and no off-target binding. The proportion loss of functional connectivity strength (PLFCS) is a new indicator for representing brain functional connectivity (FC) alteration. This study aims to estimate the relationship between the regional tau accumulation and brain FC abnormality in Alzheimer's disease (AD) and mild cognitive impairment (MCI) patients based on Florzolotau PET and fMRI. Methods: 22 NC (normal control), 31 MCI and 42 AD patients who have already been scanned with ^{18}F-Florzolotau PET were recruited in this study. (We calculated the PLFCS and standardized uptake value ratio (SUVR) of each node based on the Brainnetome atlas (BNA) template. The SUVR of 246 brain regions was calculated with the cerebellum as the reference region. Further functional connection strength (FCs), PLFCS and SUVR of each brain region were obtained in three groups for comparison.) For each patient, PLFCS and standardized uptake value ratio (SUVR) were calculated based on the Brainnetome atlas (BNA) template. These results, as well as functional connection strength (FCs), were then compared between different groups. Multiple permutation tests were used to determine the target nodes between NC and cognitive impairment (CI) groups (MCI and AD). The relationship between PLFCS and neuropsychological scores or cortical tau deposit was investigated via Pearson correlation analysis. Results: Higher PLFCS and FCs in AD and MCI groups were found compared to the NC group. The PLFCS of 129 brain regions were found to be different between NC and CI groups, and 8 of them were correlated with tau SUVR, including superior parietal lobule (MCI: $r = 0.4360$, $p = 0.0260$, AD: $r = -0.3663$, $p = 0.0280$), middle frontal gyrus (AD: MFG_R_7_2: $r = 0.4106$, $p = 0.0129$; MFG_R_7_5: $r = 0.4239$, $p = 0.0100$), inferior frontal gyrus (AD: IFG_R_6_2: $r = 0.3589$, $p = 0.0316$), precentral gyrus (AD: PrG_R_6_6: $r = 0.3493$, $p = 0.0368$), insular gyrus (AD: INS_R_6_3: $r = 0.3496$, $p = 0.0366$) and lateral occipital cortex (AD: LOcC _L_4_3: $r = -0.3433$, $p = 0.0404$). Noteworthily, the opposing relationship was found in the superior parietal lobule in the MCI and AD groups. Conclusions: Brain functional connectivity abnormality is correlated with tau pathology in AD and MCI.

Keywords: Florzolotau PET; functional connectivity; mild cognitive impairment; Alzheimer's disease

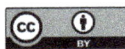

1. Introduction

Alzheimer's disease (AD) is an irreversible, devastating neurodegenerative disorder characterized by the aberrant accumulation and aggregation of amyloid plaques and neurofibrillary tangles in the brain [1]. Mild Cognitive Impairment (MCI) is identified as a prodromal phase of AD, with 10–15% conversion to dementia per year [2]. While as the most common dementia, available treatments of AD can only relieve clinical symptoms, none of the interventions are able to slow down its development. Therefore, the pathological mechanism and early diagnosis of AD have attracted increasing interest. Tau deposition and spreading are major factors of AD, which exist early in the cascade of AD etiopathogenesis and result in neuronal loss and cognitive decline [3]. Thus, it is considered an ideal target for diagnosis and novel treatments. To evaluate the pathological tau burden in vivo, a wide variety of tracers were developed based on the diverse binding targets of tau-paired helical filaments(PHFs), including quinoline derivatives and benzimidazole pyrimidine derivatives [4–8]. Since the first tau radioligand, ^{18}F-FDDNP, was developed, a variety of tracers have been synthesized and have demonstrated promising results in the clinical evaluation of tau deposition. However, the first-generation tau tracers showed several limitations, including high binding affinity in the deep brain nucleus, where pathological studies did not show a high density of tangles in AD and "off-target" binding to monoamine oxidase B (MAO-B). Compared with them, the second-generation tau tracers showed lower "off-target" binding and improved affinity and selectivity in tau aggregates [9], which enhanced the detection of the affected subregions in the early phase of AD. Several clinical trials have verified that the distribution of tau tracers is related to post-mortem neuropathology in primary tauopathies [10], and the binding of tracers is associated with cognitive performance in AD patients [10]. Moreover, tau PET imaging can contribute to further elaboration on the relationship between tau accumulation and other biomarkers or clinical symptoms.

Brain functional connectivity (FC) is able to evaluate the spatiotemporal association between distinct cerebral cortical regions, which can offer novel perspectives on functional brain disruption and other abnormalities caused by neuropathies [11]. In several neurodegenerative diseases, neuropathology and atrophy are most prominent in nodes with dense connections (usually referred to as 'hubs') [12], both at the structural [13] and functional levels [14]. Abnormal functional connectivity strength (FCs) in AD and its preclinical stages have been estimated via resting-state functional magnetic resonance imaging (rs-fMRI) in previous studies [15,16]. Several studies were launched to evaluate the correlation between functional abnormality and tau deposition in AD and its preclinical stages [17–20]. Combined with tau positron emission tomography (PET) scan, studies provided evidence that tau toxicity can influence neuronal activity and synaptic plasticity and lead to the disruption of FC. For instance, Hansson et al. proposed that there were spatial correspondences between major functional networks and regional pathological tau accumulation [21,22]. Cope et al. has demonstrated that tau burden is correlated with a higher graph theoretical index of functional connectivity evaluated in AD [22]. Specifically, the proportion loss of functional connectivity strength (PLFCS) was assessed, which ensured that the results did not issue from the bias introduced by proportionate thresholding. This index is associated with weighted degree, while it is more subject to fMRI signal-to-noise ratio limitations in comparison to traditional FC metrics. Previous studies showed that the PLFCS is a relatively new index of research, and it holds possibilities in revealing the brain function change in AD and other neurodegenerative diseases [23–25]. However, all these studies were launched with the use of first-generation tau tracers.

In this study, we used the second-generation tau radiotracer ^{18}F-Florzolotau to evaluate the relationship between the abnormal FC (including functional connection strength and PLFCS) and tau deposition, as well as neuropsychological scores in AD and MCI, and further explored the role of tau accumulation in the FC abnormality during AD disease progression.

2. Materials and Methods
2.1. Participants

We prospectively recruited 36 AD patients, 26 MCI patients and 22 NC subjects who underwent Florzolotau PET scanning in Huashan Hospital affiliated with Fudan University in this study. Besides Florzolotau PET, T1-weighted structural MRI and fMRI scanning was also needed for each subject. All participants needed to be over 55 years and fulfill the following research criteria: (1) AD patients have completed an ^{18}F-AV45 PET scan and been characterized as amyloid PET-positive; (2) subjects have conducted The Mini-Mental State Examination (MMSE) and Clinical Dementia Rating–Sum of Boxes (CDR-SB) test by experienced neurologists from Huashan hospital; (3) NCs had an MMSE score of 24 or greater, and no history of cognitive impairment, mental disorders, neurological diseases or brain trauma. Clinically probable AD was diagnosed with the 2011 NIA-AA guidelines [24], and the diagnosis of MCI required to meet Petersen's criteria [26]; (4) dementia caused by other reasons needs to be excluded.

This study was approved by the Institutional Review Board of Huashan Hospital (HIRB) (no. 2018-363). All subjects or a legally responsible relative gave written informed consent before the study.

2.2. Acquisition Protocol

All subjects withdrew cognitive enhancing and psychotropic medicine for at least 12 h before clinical assessment and each imaging acquisition. Participants underwent T1-weighted structural MRI and rs-fMRI on a 3.0T horizontal magnet (Discovery MR750; GE Medical Systems, Milwaukee, WI) and a T1 MRI image was acquired with FOV = 25.6 cm, matrix = $256 \times 256 \times 152$, slice thickness = 1 mm, repetition time (TR) = 8.2 ms, echo time (TE) = 3.2 ms, flip angle= 12°. The Rs-fMRI scans were performed with the following parameters: FOV = 24 cm, slice thickness = 3 mm, TR = 8800 ms, TE = 145 ms, flip angle = 77°. PET data were obtained by the use of a Siemens mCT Flow PET/CT (Siemens, Erlangen, Germany) in a PET center, Huashan Hospital, in the three-dimensional (3D) mode. ^{18}F-Florzolotau PET imaging was performed for 20 minutes, 90–110 minutes after 370 MBq ^{18}F-Florzolotau was intravenously injected. Images were corrected by the mode of CT attenuation correction, and the reconstruction was performed with the ordered subset expectation maximization (OSEM) method.

2.3. Data Pre-Processing

Rs-fMRI data were processed with the use of DPARSF (http://www.rfmri.org/DPARSF, accessed on 10 January 2022). First, in order to stabilize the initial signal and allow individuals to acclimate to the environment, the first 10 volumes were discarded. Volumes remaining according to acquisition time were corrected and realigned to the head movement of the first volume, and mean signals from white matter (WM), cerebrospinal fluid (CSF) and Friston-24 head motion parameters were regressed out. Then, the T1 images were registered with the fMRI at the individual level. The segmented T1 images were spatially normalized based on the standard Montreal Neurological Institute (MNI) brain space. All images were resampled into $3 \times 3 \times 3$ mm^3 voxels. Finally, the linear drift and corrections for white matter, CSF signals, six head movement parameters and band-pass filters (0.01–0.08 Hz) of the fMRI data were removed. Smoothing was based on a 4 mm full-width half-height (EWHM) filter.

PET data were processed using Statistical Parametric Mapping 12 (the Wellcome Department of Neurology, London, UK) package. First, PET images were registered based on the T1 images of the corresponding subjects. Second, the gray matter (GM) tissue probability map from segmented T1 images was registered. Then, based on the MNI standard space, the GM map was registered using nonlinear transformation parameters. The registered PET images were also spatially normalized using the same transformation parameters and were then resampled into $2 \times 2 \times 2$ mm^3 voxels. Finally, PET was smoothed based on an 8 mm full-width half-height filter.

2.4. Brain Network Analysis

2.4.1. Functional Connection Strength

The Brainnetome atlas (BNA) contains 246 brain regions of the bilateral hemispheres (available at http://atlas.brainnetome.org/, last accessed on 31 August 2022). Each brain region was treated as a node used for network analysis based on Pearson's correlation to estimate time-resolved fMRI connectivity. Thus, each subject obtained a 246 × 246 association matrix and Fisher z-transform. The individual connection strength of each node was quantified by the sum of the absolute values of the associated value between the node and other nodes, then the connection strength of the node was defined as the average value of the individual connection strength for each diagnostic group.

2.4.2. Proportional Loss of Connectional Strength

The individual-level PLFCS in the disease group was defined as the difference in connectivity strength from the normal control group and was scaled based on the baseline group. The value of PLFCS was calculated as equation (1):

$$\text{Loss}_i = \frac{\mu_i - \sigma}{\sigma} \qquad (1)$$

where μ_i is the connection strength of each node. σ is the average connection strength of all nodes in the baseline [23,27].

2.5. Semi-Quantitative ROI-Based PET Analyses

The entire cerebellum was selected as the reference region for calculating the normalized uptake value ratios (SUVRs) in 246 brain regions based on PET images. Then, for comparison with functional connection strength, the group-averaged SUVR of each brain region was obtained.

2.6. Comparison of PLFCS along AD Spectrum

Except for these three groups, we define the cognitive impairment (CI) group as the sum total of AD and MCI patients. To determine robust PLFCS biomarkers, we performed a two-sample t-test for PLFCS in the 246 brain regions of the NC and the CI group. We considered brain regions with significant differences ($p < 0.05$) as potential biomarkers and presented them using boxplots.

2.7. Correlation between Proportional Loss and Clinical Scales

We first checked the relationship between the PLFCS and functional connection strength (un-transformed) of 246 brain regions in the disease groups to evaluate whether brain regions with high connection strength were vulnerable to the effect of neuropathology, based on our hypotheses that the proportionate vulnerability of these regions can reflect the progression of neurodegeneration. It was expected that regions with relatively higher connection strength tend to lose more. Therefore, we performed a correlation analysis between the averaged proportional loss of hub regions and cognitive level in the disease groups, where the cognitive level was reflected by clinical scales of MMSE and CDR-SB.

2.8. Statistical Analysis

A two-sample t-test was performed for continuous variables comparison, and the χ test was used for the between-group differences of categorical variables. Correlations between fMRI data and tau levels and clinical scales were assessed for each diagnostic group based on Pearson correlation. We analyzed differences of clinical variates among three groups with the use of univariate analysis of variance (ANOVA) and Bonferroni's post hoc analysis or Dunn's multiple test on account of homogeneity of variance. All statistical analyses were performed on the SPSS 19.0 platform, and $p < 0.05$ was considered significant.

3. Results

3.1. Demographic

The subject's demographics and scores of cognitive examination are displayed in Table 1. The average age of the MCI group was older than NC and AD, whereas the difference between NC and AD subjects was not statistically significant (p = 0.226). Lower MMSE and higher CDR-SB scores were observed in AD and MCI than NC group. No differences in education years were found among the three groups.

Table 1. Demographic information and scores of cognitive examinations.

Group	Number	Gender (Male/Female)	Age of Scanning	Education	MMSE	CDR-SB
NC	22	8/14	56.95 ± 7.01	11.27 ± 3.92	28.23 ± 1.41	0.00 ± 0.00
MCI	26	6/20	70.38 ± 8.47	10.27 ± 3.29	25.53 ± 1.70	4.46 ± 1.46
AD	36	14/22	60.94 ± 10.13	9.86 ± 3.86	16.00 ± 6.29	8.68 ± 3.96
p	-	0.217 [a]	<0.001 [b]	0.358 [b]	<0.001 [c]	<0.001 [b]

[a] Chi-square test. [b] One-way ANOVA test with Bonferroni's multiple comparison test. [c] ANOVA test with Dunn's multiple comparison test. p < 0.05 was considered as significant. p-values are given for the comparisons among the three groups. Data are presented as mean ± standard deviation. AD, Alzheimer's disease; CDR-SB, Clinical Dementia Rating–Sum of Boxes; NC, normal control subjects; MCI, patients with mild cognitive impairment; MMSE, Mini-Mental State Examination.

3.2. Results of PLFCS and Tau Level

Higher FCs and PLFCS were found in the MCI and AD groups than in the NC group, and differences were not found between the AD and MCI groups (FCs: p = 0.971, Figure 1a; PLFCS: p = 0.652, Figure 1b). Higher globally averaged tau SUVR was found in the AD group than in the MCI and NC groups, and differences were not found between the NC and MCI groups (p = 0.887, Figure 1c).

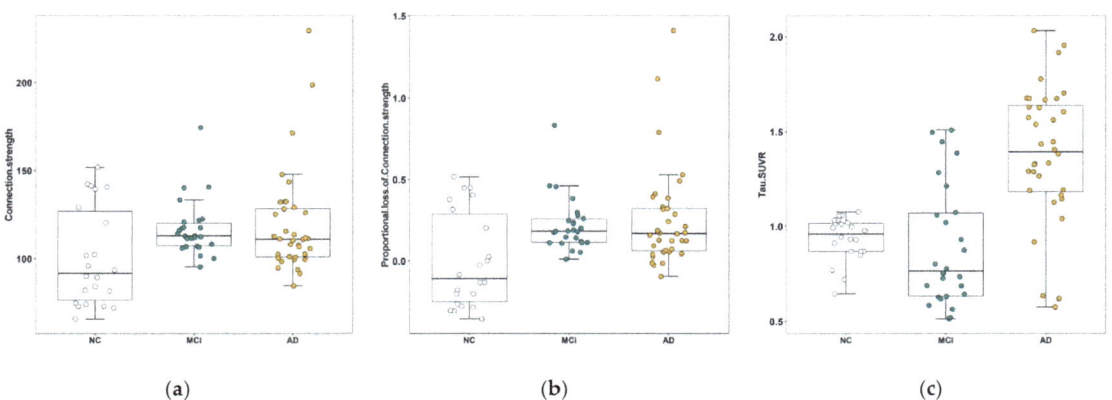

Figure 1. Comparison of connection strength, PLFCS and tau SUVR between the three groups. (**a**) The global FCs of NC, MCI and AD groups. (**b**) The comparison of global PLFCS between NC, MCI and AD groups. (**c**) The comparison of global tau SUVR between the NC, MCI and AD groups. Abbreviations: NC, normal control; MCI, mild cognitive impairment; AD, Alzheimer's disease.

We found differences in the PLFCS level between the NC and CI groups in 129 brain regions and further analyzed the correlation between PLFCS and tau SUVR in these regions. Brain regions with significant correlation are shown in Table 2 and Figure 2, including superior parietal lobule (MCI: r = 0.4360, p = 0.0260, AD: r = −0.3663, p = 0.0280), middle frontal gyrus (AD: MFG_R_7_2: r = 0.4106, p = 0.0129; MFG_R_7_5: r = 0.4239, p = 0.0100), inferior frontal gyrus (AD: IFG_R_6_2: r = 0.3589, p = 0.0316), precentral gyrus (AD: PrG_R_6_6: r = 0.3493, p = 0.0368), insular gyrus (AD: INS_R_6_3: r = 0.3496, p = 0.0366) and lateral occipital cortex (AD: LOcC_L_4_3: $r = -0.3433$, $p = 0.0404$). Noteworthily, the inverse relationship was found in the superior parietal lobule in the MCI and AD groups. Further, we analyzed the relationship between SUVR/PLFCS and clinical scores, and no significant correlation was found.

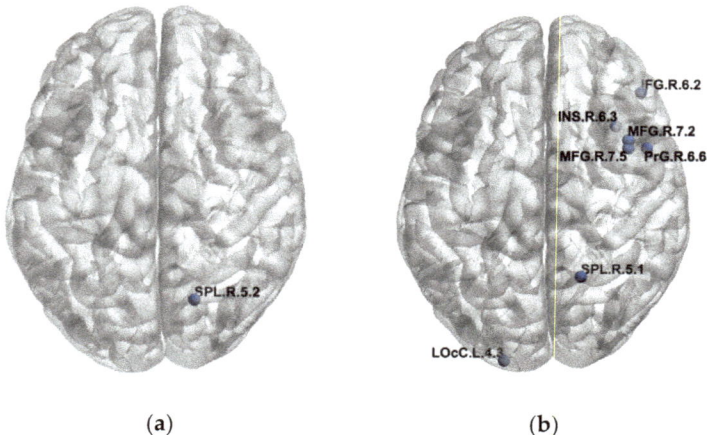

Figure 2. Detailed brain regions with significant correlation of FCs/PLFCS and tau SUVR. (**a**) Brain regions with significant correlation of FCs/PLFCS and tau SUVR in the MCI group. (**b**) Brain regions with significant correlation of FCs/PLFCS and tau SUVR in the AD group.

3.3. Correlation of FC and PLFCS

The correlation between the group-averaged FCs and PLFCS of the cerebral cortex of the MCI and AD groups with that of the NC group are shown in Figure 2. We found that brain regions with higher functional connectivity in normal control subjects lost the larger proportion of connection strength in MCI ($r = -0.7736$, $p < 0.0001$, Figure 3a) and AD ($r = -0.7999$, $p < 0.0001$, Figure 3b).

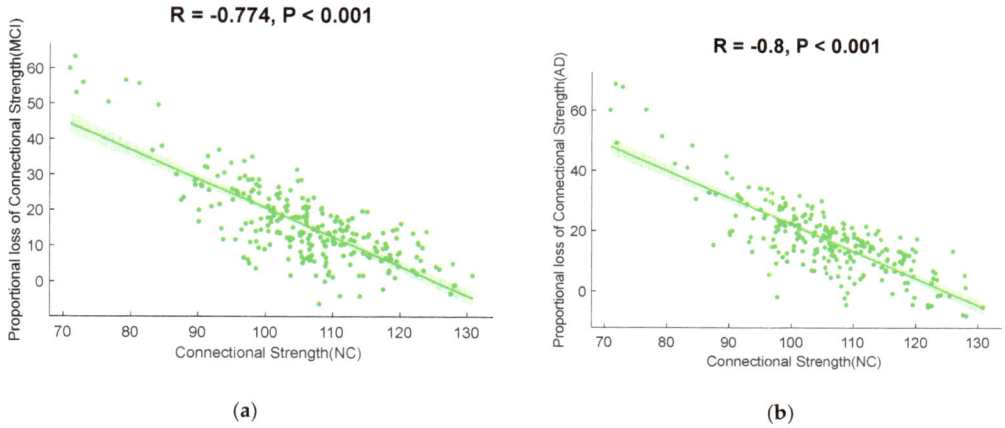

Figure 3. Scatterplots illustrating the relationship between the connectional strength in normal controls and PLFCS in disease groups. (**a**) The correlation between the connectional strength in normal controls and the PLFCS in MCI subjects. (**b**) The correlation between the connectional strength in normal controls and PLFCS in AD subjects.

Table 2. Brain regions with significant correlation of FCs/PLFCS and tau SUVR.

				MCI						
Lobe	Gyrus	Left and Right Hemispheres	Label ID.L	Label ID.R	Modified Cyto-Architectonic	lh.MNI (X, Y, Z)	rh.MNI (X, Y, Z)	R(FCs and Tau SUVR)	P (FCs and tau SUVR)	R (PLFCS and Tau SUVR)	P (PLFCS and Tau SUVR)
Parietal lobe	SPL, superior parietal lobule	SPL_R_5_2		128	A7c, caudal area 7	−15, −71, 52	19, −69, 54	0.4332	0.0271	0.4360	0.0260
				AD							
Lobe	Gyrus	Left and Right Hemispheres	Label ID.L	Label ID.R	Modified Cyto-Architectonic	lh.MNI (X,Y,Z)	rh.MNI (X,Y,Z)	R (FCs and Tau SUVR)	P (FCs and Tau SUVR)	R (PLFCS and Tau SUVR)	P (PLFCS and Tau SUVR)
Frontal lobe	MFG, middle frontal gyrus	MFG_R_7_2		18	IFJ, inferior frontal junction	−42, 13, 36	42, 11, 39	0.4159	0.0116	0.4106	0.0129
	MFG, middle frontal gyrus	MFG_R_7_5		24	A8vl, ventrolateral area 8	−33, 23, 45	42, 27, 39	0.4214	0.0105	0.4239	0.0100
	IFG, inferior frontal gyrus	IFG_R_6_2		32	IFS, inferior frontal sulcus	−47, 32, 14	48, 35, 13	0.3656	0.0283	0.3589	0.0316
	PrG, precentral gyrus	PrG_R_6_6		64	A6cvl, caudal ventrolateral area 6	−49, 5, 30	51, 7, 30	0.3420	0.0412	0.3493	0.0368
Parietal lobe	SPL, superior parietal lobule	SPL_R_5_1		126	A7r, rostral area 7	−16, −60, 63	19, −57, 65	−0.3624	0.0299	−0.3663	0.0280
Insular lobe	INS, insular gyrus	INS_R_6_3		168	dIa, dorsal agranular insula	−34, 18, 1	36, 18, 1	0.3321	0.0478	0.3496	0.0366
Occipital lobe	LOcC, lateral occipital cortex	LOcC_L_4_3	203		OPC, occipital polar cortex	−18, −99, 2	22, −97, 4	−0.3443	0.0397	−0.3432	0.0404

4. Discussion

The study aimed to investigate the neurophysiological FC abnormality in AD and MCI and its relationship with tau burden. We found higher PLFCS and functional connection strength in the AD and MCI groups compared to NCs. Global tau SUVR of the AD group was higher than that of the NC group, but no difference was found between the AD and MCI groups. Significant relationships between the FCs of NC groups and the PLFCS of disease groups were observed, which strongly supported the hypotheses that brain regions with relatively higher functional connectivity would be more vulnerable to tau accumulation in neurodegeneration [28]. PLFCS of several brain regions were found to be different between the NC and CI groups, and some of them were correlated with tau SUVR, including superior parietal lobule, middle frontal gyrus, inferior frontal gyrus, precentral gyrus, insular gyrus and lateral occipital cortex. Notably, relationships were found in the superior parietal lobule in both MCI and AD groups.

Consistent with our results, Cho et al. found that ^{18}F-flortaucipir SUVR increased in the superior parietal cortex, and the change was correlated with the progression of diffuse volume atrophy during a 2-year-follow-up in the MCI group, and the correlation pattern with clinical scores was not included [29]. The cortical thickness of the superior parietal lobule was found to be associated with mild symptoms and signs of cognitive impairment in AD [30], indicating that the functional and structural abnormality in the superior parietal lobule were correlated with disease progression but did not directly influence the cognitive performance of patients. Strikingly, in the AD group, we found that PLFCS was negatively correlated with tau SUVR, and in MCI, this relationship was inversed, with the value of PLFCS increasing in line with the tau level. This may be a compensatory phenomenon. The cognitive function of healthy aging depends on maintaining connectivity within and between large-scale networks [31], which can increase the fault tolerance of the network to disease [32]. By the time AD pathology is sufficiently advanced to trigger the clinical signs of MCI, tau has generally already emerged to some degree throughout the neocortex [33], thus the functional connections of some nodes are strengthened to balance the weakening of those strongest functional connections, which are caused by tau pathology [34].

We found a negative relationship between FCs/PLFCS and the tau level in the occipital and parietal lobes and a positive relationship in the frontal lobe; however, both tau and FCs/PLFCS were not associated with cognitive function (evaluated by MMSE and CDR-SB) in these brain regions. Several studies have reported the same fronto-occipital functional alteration pattern and demonstrated that this change was associated with cognition and tau level [33–36], suggesting a reconstructed brain network, including further disconnection and isolation in parietal and occipital nodes and compensatory frontal network with the progression of AD. Our PLFCS findings not only consolidated those results but also indicated that the local tau accumulation might be a reason for the network's alteration in AD progression, and there was no interactive effect of the tau burden with functional connectivity alteration on cognitive function. To our knowledge, this is the first time these have been verified with a second tau PET tracer, and the results are consistent with previous studies, which show convincing evidence of the value of second-generation tau tracers Florzolotau in studies on AD continuum.

Though the average level of PLFCS in AD subjects was prominently higher than that of NCs, the PLFCS value cannot distinguish AD from MCI. Considering that both aging and neurodegeneration contribute to the disruption of the functional network, the higher PLFCS level in the MCI group may result from their older age [37]. A previous study found that it was age-related that the connectivity in the MCI group was significantly stronger than that in the NC group [38]. During the aging and memory deficit process, an evident reduction in the connection strength was demonstrated as attributed to factors such as the massive loss of neurons and synapses during the development of aging and AD [9].

Besides the regions shown in the current study, several studies have also reported that regional connectivity alteration might be a potential biomarker of the AD continuum and relate to proteinopathies. Li et al. found that FCs decreased in the left MTG of MCI patients, particularly in the vascular MCI (VaMCI) [39]. Our previous study performed individually specified PLFCS to quantitatively characterize the decrease degree and the PLFCS of the left middle temporal gyrus that yielded a powerful diagnostic efficacy of 80% for categorizing SCD from NC. Moreover, significant gray matter volume reductions, altered FC pattern and density, together with severely decreased amplitude of low-frequency fluctuation in the left MTG have been reported in previous studies on MCI [40–43]. These findings indicated that the MTG was a crucial network node with rich connections, and it could be a promising target in studies of the AD continuum. In addition to MTG, other regional connectome alterations such as hippocampal connectivity [17] and frontoparietal control network hubs [43] were also reported on MCI and AD, and some were proven to be related to tau pathology in disease progression [44]. Therefore, other FC assessments would be used to estimate the functional abnormality and its relationship with tau burden, and additional regional connectome influenced by cognition impairment-related pathological alterations would be analyzed in further studies, which might offer new insights into the pathological interpretation of the relationship between tau accumulation and the functional connectivity and find more potential biomarkers in the AD continuum.

This study had several shortcomings. First, the sample size was relatively small and statistical differences in age and MMSE scores were found between groups, which limited our interpretation of causality. Secondly, the AD group included patients with different severity, which might influence the uptake levels of Florzolotau in brain regions and further result in different relationships with PLFCS. Meanwhile, only the MMSE and CDR-SB scores were used to estimate the cognitive function of AD and MCI patients. More subdomain evaluations, such as memory, executive function and others, are needed so that we can evaluate the cognitive changes in AD patients more accurately.

5. Conclusions

In summary, we have shown the negative relationship between FCs/PLFCS and tau level in the occipital and parietal lobes and a positive relationship in the frontal lobe, suggesting that the local tau accumulation might be a reason for the functional alteration and network reconstruction during the AD progression. An inverse relationship between PLFCS and tau SUVR in SPL was found in the MCI and AD groups, indicating that a compensatory functional strengthening may exist in some nodes in response to the regional tau toxicity. These findings provide preliminary evidence that brain FC alteration is associated with tau pathology in AD and its prodromal stage and motivates the exploration of AD physiopathology with the combination of rs-fMRI and PET imaging with a second-generation tau tracer.

Author Contributions: Conceptualization, H.Z. and J.J.; Data Curation, Z.J. and Z.L.; Writing—Original Draft Preparation, Z.J., Z.L., J.L., F.J., H.L., W.B., M.L., Q.Z., J.J. and H.Z.; Writing—Review and Editing, Z.J., Z.L., J.L., F.J., H.L., W.B., M.L., P.W., Y.G., Q.Z., J.J., H.Z. and C.Z.; Supervision, H.Z., J.J. and C.Z.; Figures, Z.J. and Z.L.; Funding Acquisition, H.Z., J.J. and C.Z.; All authors have read and agreed to the published version of the manuscript.

Funding: This work is supported by National Natural Science Foundation of China (81901367, 82021002, 81971641 and 81671239), the Open Program of Nuclear Medicine and Molecular Imaging Key Laboratory of Sichuan Province (HYX21002), the Research project of Shanghai Health Commission (2020YJZX0111), the Clinical Research Plan of SHDC (SHDC2020CR1038B), Science and Technology Innovation 2030 Major Projects (2022ZD0211600) and the Shanghai Medical Center New Star Young Medical Talents Training Funding Program.

Institutional Review Board Statement: Not applicable.

Informed Consent Statement: Not applicable.

Data Availability Statement: Not applicable.

Acknowledgments: We thank all the patients and family members who participated in the study. We are grateful to APRINOIA Therapeutics for the provision of the ^{18}F-Florzolotau precursor.

Conflicts of Interest: The authors declare no conflict of interest. The funders had no role in the study's design, in the collection, analyses, or interpretation of data, in the writing of the manuscript, or in the decision to publish the results.

References

1. Zhang, Z.; Yang, X.; Song, Y.Q.; Tu, J. Autophagy in Alzheimer's disease pathogenesis: Therapeutic potential and future perspectives. *Ageing Res. Rev.* **2021**, *72*, 101464. [CrossRef] [PubMed]
2. Risacher, S.L.; Saykin, A.J. Neuroimaging in aging and neurologic diseases. *Handb. Clin. Neurol.* **2019**, *167*, 191–227.
3. Jack, C.R., Jr.; Knopman, D.S.; Jagust, W.J.; Shaw, L.M.; Aisen, P.S.; Weiner, M.W.; Petersen, R.C.; Trojanowski, J.Q. Hypothetical model of dynamic biomarkers of the Alzheimer's pathological cascade. *Lancet Neurol.* **2010**, *9*, 119–128. [CrossRef]
4. Kang, J.M.; Lee, S.Y.; Seo, S.; Jeong, H.J.; Woo, S.H.; Lee, H.; Lee, Y.B.; Yeon, B.K.; Shin, D.H.; Park, K.H.; et al. Tau positron emission tomography using [^{18}F]THK$_{5351}$ and cerebral glucose hypometabolism in Alzheimer's disease. *Neurobiol. Aging* **2017**, *59*, 210–219. [CrossRef] [PubMed]
5. Kitamura, S.; Shimada, H.; Niwa, F.; Endo, H.; Shinotoh, H.; Takahata, K.; Kubota, M.; Takado, Y.; Hirano, S.; Kimura, Y.; et al. Tau-induced focal neurotoxicity and network disruption related to apathy in Alzheimer's disease. *J. Neurol. Neurosurg. Psychiatry* **2018**, *89*, 1208–1214. [CrossRef] [PubMed]
6. Landau, S.M.; Fero, A.; Baker, S.L.; Koeppe, R.; Mintun, M.; Chen, K.; Reiman, E.M.; Jagust, W.J. Measurement of longitudinal β-amyloid change with ^{18}F-florbetapir PET and standardized uptake value ratios. *J. Nucl. Med.* **2015**, *56*, 567–574. [CrossRef] [PubMed]
7. Leuzy, A.; Chiotis, K.; Lemoine, L.; Gillberg, P.G.; Almkvist, O.; Rodriguez-Vieitez, E.; Nordberg, A. Tau PET imaging in neurodegenerative tauopathies-still a challenge. *Mol. Psychiatry* **2019**, *24*, 1112–1134. [CrossRef] [PubMed]
8. Lohith, T.G.; Bennacef, I.; Vandenberghe, R.; Vandenbulcke, M.; Salinas, C.A.; Declercq, R.; Reynders, T.; Telan-Choing, N.F.; Riffel, K.; Celen, S.; et al. Brain imaging of Alzheimer dementia patients and elderly controls with ^{18}F-MK-6240, a PET tracer targeting neurofibrillary tangles. *J. Nucl. Med.* **2019**, *60*, 107–114. [CrossRef]
9. Lu, J.; Bao, W.; Li, M.; Li, L.; Zhang, Z.; Alberts, I.; Brendel, M.; Cumming, P.; Lu, H.; Xiao, Z.; et al. Associations of [^{18}F]-APN-1607 Tau PET Binding in the Brain of Alzheimer's Disease Patients With Cognition and Glucose Metabolism. *Front. Neurosci.* **2020**, *14*, 604. [CrossRef] [PubMed]
10. Smith, R.; Puschmann, A.; Schöll, M.; Ohlsson, T.; van Swieten, J.; Honer, M.; Englund, E.; Hansson, O. ^{18}F-AV-1451 tau PET imaging correlates strongly with tau neuropathology in MAPT mutation carriers. *Brain* **2016**, *139*, 2372–2379. [CrossRef]
11. Buckner, R.L.; Sepulcre, J.; Talukdar, T.; Krienen, F.M.; Liu, H.; Hedden, T.; Andrews-Hanna, J.R.; Sperling, R.A.; Johnson, K.A. Cortical hubs revealed by intrinsic functional connectivity: Mapping, assessment of stability, and relation to Alzheimer's disease. *J. Neurosci.* **2009**, *29*, 1860–1873. [CrossRef]
12. Crossley, N.A.; Mechelli, A.; Scott, J.; Carletti, F.; Fox, P.T.; McGuire, P.; Bullmore, E.T. The hubs of the human connectome are generally implicated in the anatomy of brain disorders. *Brain* **2014**, *137 Pt 8*, 2382–2395. [CrossRef] [PubMed]
13. Dai, Z.; Yan, C.; Li, K.; Wang, Z.; Wang, J.; Cao, M.; Lin, Q.; Shu, N.; Xia, M.; Bi, Y.; et al. Identifying and mapping connectivity patterns of brain network hubs in Alzheimer's disease. *Cereb. Cortex* **2015**, *25*, 3723–3742. [CrossRef]
14. Li, H.; Gao, S.; Jia, X.; Jiang, T.; Li, K. Distinctive Alterations of Functional Connectivity Strength between Vascular and Amnestic Mild Cognitive Impairment. *Neural Plast.* **2021**, *2021*, 8812490. [CrossRef] [PubMed]
15. Zhu, Q.; Wang, Y.; Zhuo, C.; Xu, Q.; Yao, Y.; Liu, Z.; Li, Y.; Sun, Z.; Wang, J.; Lv, M.; et al. Classification of Alzheimer's Disease Based on Abnormal Hippocampal Functional Connectivity and Machine Learning. *Front. Aging Neurosci.* **2022**, *14*, 754334. [CrossRef] [PubMed]
16. Fu, L.; Zhou, Z.; Liu, L.; Zhang, J.; Xie, H.; Zhang, X.; Zhu, M.; Wang, R. Functional Abnormality Associated with Tau Deposition in Alzheimer's Disease—A Hybrid Positron Emission Tomography/MRI Study. *Front. Aging Neurosci.* **2021**, *13*, 758053. [CrossRef] [PubMed]
17. Adams, J.N.; Maass, A.; Harrison, T.M.; Baker, S.L.; Jagust, W.J. Cortical tau deposition follows patterns of entorhinal functional connectivity in aging. *eLife* **2019**, *8*, e49132. [CrossRef] [PubMed]
18. Hansson, O.; Grothe, M.J.; Strandberg, T.O.; Ohlsson, T.; Hägerström, D.; Jögi, J.; Smith, R.; Schöll, M. Tau Pathology Distribution in Alzheimer's disease Corresponds Differentially to Cognition-Relevant Functional Brain Networks. *Front. Neurosci.* **2017**, *11*, 167. [CrossRef] [PubMed]
19. Hoenig, M.C.; Bischof, G.N.; Seemiller, J.; Hammes, J.; Kukolja, J.; Onur, Ö.A.; Jessen, F.; Fliessbach, K.; Neumaier, B.; Fink, G.R.; et al. Networks of tau distribution in Alzheimer's disease. *Brain* **2018**, *141*, 568–581. [CrossRef] [PubMed]
20. Franzmeier, N.; Neitzel, J.; Rubinski, A.; Smith, R.; Strandberg, O.; Ossenkoppele, R.; Hansson, O.; Ewers, M.; Alzheimer's Disease Neuroimaging Initiative (ADNI). Functional brain architecture is associated with the rate of tau accumulation in Alzheimer's disease. *Nat. Commun.* **2020**, *11*, 347. [CrossRef] [PubMed]

21. Franzmeier, N.; Rubinski, A.; Neitzel, J.; Kim, Y.; Damm, A.; Na, D.L.; Kim, H.J.; Lyoo, C.H.; Cho, H.; Finsterwalder, S.; et al. Functional connectivity associated with tau levels in ageing. Alzheimer's, and small vessel disease. *Brain* 2019, *142*, 1093–1107. [CrossRef]
22. Cope, T.E.; Rittman, T.; Borchert, R.J.; Jones, P.S.; Vatansever, D.; Allinson, K.; Passamonti, L.; Rodriguez, P.V.; Bevan-Jones, W.R.; O'Brien, J.T.; et al. Tau burden and the functional connectome in Alzheimer's disease and progressive supranuclear palsy. *Brain* 2018, *141*, 550–567. [CrossRef] [PubMed]
23. Achard, S.; Delon-Martin, C.; Vértes, P.E.; Renard, F.; Schenck, M.; Schneider, F.; Heinrich, C.; Kremer, S.; Bullmore, E.T. Hubs of brain functional networks are radically reorganized in comatose patients. *Proc. Natl. Acad. Sci. USA* 2012, *109*, 20608–20613. [CrossRef] [PubMed]
24. Petersen, R.C. Mild cognitive impairment as a diagnostic entity. *J. Intern. Med.* 2004, *256*, 183–194. [CrossRef] [PubMed]
25. McKhann, G.M.; Knopman, D.S.; Chertkow, H.; Hyman, B.T.; Jack, C.R., Jr.; Kawas, C.H.; Klunk, W.E.; Koroshetz, W.J.; Manly, J.J.; Mayeux, R.; et al. The diagnosis of dementia due to Alzheimer'sdisease: Recommendations from the National Institute on Aging-Alzheimer's Association workgroups on diagnostic guidelines for Alzheimer's disease. *Alzheimer's Dement.* 2011, *7*, 263–269. [CrossRef] [PubMed]
26. Rittman, T.; Rubinov, M.; Vértes, P.E.; Patel, A.X.; Ginestet, C.E.; Ghosh, B.C.P.; Barker, R.A.; Spillantini, M.G.; Bullmore, E.T.; Rowe, J.B. Regional expression of the MAPT gene is associated with loss of hubs in brain networks and cognitive impairment in Parkinson disease and progressive supranuclear palsy. *Neurobiol. Aging* 2016, *48*, 153–160. [CrossRef]
27. Cho, H.; Choi, J.Y.; Lee, H.S.; Lee, J.H.; Ryu, Y.H.; Lee, M.S.; Jack, C.R., Jr.; Lyoo, C.H. Progressive Tau Accumulation in Alzheimer Disease: 2-Year Follow-up Study. *J. Nucl. Med.* 2019, *60*, 1611–1621. [CrossRef] [PubMed]
28. Bakkour, A.; Morris, J.C.; Dickerson, B.C. The cortical signature of prodromal AD: Regional thinning predicts mild AD dementia. *Neurology* 2009, *72*, 1048–1055. [CrossRef] [PubMed]
29. Tsvetanov, K.A.; Henson, R.N.; Tyler, L.K.; Razi, A.; Geerligs, L.; Ham, T.E.; Rowe, J.B.; Cambridge Centre for Ageing and Neuroscience. Extrinsic and Intrinsic Brain Network Connectivity Maintains Cognition across the Lifespan Despite Accelerated Decay of Regional Brain Activation. *J. Neurosci.* 2016, *36*, 3115–3126. [CrossRef] [PubMed]
30. Strogatz, S.H. Exploring complex networks. *Nature* 2001, *410*, 268–276. [CrossRef]
31. Markesbery, W.R. Neuropathologic alterations in mild cognitive impairment: A review. *J. Alzheimer's Dis.* 2010, *19*, 221–228. [CrossRef] [PubMed]
32. Adriaanse, S.M.; Wink, A.M.; Tijms, B.M.; Ossenkoppele, R.; Verfaillie, S.C.; Lammertsma, A.A.; Boellaard, R.; Scheltens, P.; van Berckel, B.N.; Barkhof, F. The Association of Glucose Metabolism and Eigenvector Centrality in Alzheimer's Disease. *Brain Connect.* 2016, *6*, 1–8. [CrossRef] [PubMed]
33. Luo, X.; Qiu, T.; Jia, Y.; Huang, P.; Xu, X.; Yu, X.; Shen, Z.; Jiaerken, Y.; Guan, X.; Zhou, J.; et al. ADNI Intrinsic functional connectivity alterations in cognitively intact elderly APOE ε4 carriers measured by eigenvector centrality mapping are related to cognition and CSF biomarkers: A preliminary study. *Brain Imaging Behav.* 2017, *11*, 1290–1301. [CrossRef] [PubMed]
34. Ossenkoppele, R.; van der Flier, W.M.; Zwan, M.D.; Adriaanse, S.F.; Boellaard, R.; Windhorst, A.D.; Barkhof, F.; Lammertsma, A.A.; Scheltens, P.; van Berckel, B.N. Differential effect of APOE genotype on amyloid load and glucose metabolism in AD dementia. *Neurology* 2013, *80*, 359–365. [CrossRef]
35. Binnewijzend, M.A.; Adriaanse, S.M.; Van der Flier, W.M.; Teunissen, C.E.; de Munck, J.C.; Stam, C.J.; Scheltens, P.; van Berckel, B.N.; Barkhof, F.; Wink, A.M. Brain network alterations in Alzheimer's disease measured by eigenvector centrality in fMRI are related to cognition and CSF biomarkers. *Hum. Brain Mapp.* 2014, *35*, 2383–2393. [CrossRef] [PubMed]
36. Courtney, S.M.; Hinault, T. When the time is right: Temporal dynamics of brain activity in healthy aging and dementia. *Prog. Neurobiol.* 2021, *203*, 102076. [CrossRef] [PubMed]
37. Yang, Z.; Caldwell, J.Z.K.; Cummings, J.L.; Ritter, A.; Kinney, J.W.; Cordes, D. Alzheimer's Disease Neuroimaging Initiative (ADNI). Sex Modulates the Pathological Aging Effect on Caudate Functional Connectivity in Mild Cognitive Impairment. *Front. Psychiatry* 2022, *13*, 804168. [PubMed]
38. Li, M.; Zheng, G.; Zheng, Y.; Xiong, Z.; Xia, R.; Zhou, W.; Wang, Q.; Liang, S.; Tao, J.; Chen, L. Alterations in resting-state functional connectivity of the default mode network in amnestic mild cognitive impairment: An fMRI study. *BMC Med. Imaging* 2017, *17*, 48. [CrossRef]
39. Stebbins, G.T.; Nyenhuis, D.L.; Wang, C.; Cox, J.L.; Freels, S.; Bangen, K.; deToledo-Morrell, L.; Sripathirathan, K.; Moseley, M.; Turner, D.A.; et al. Gray matter atrophy in patients with ischemic stroke with cognitive impairment. *Stroke* 2008, *39*, 785–793. [CrossRef]
40. Li, K.; Chan, W.; Doody, R.S.; Quinn, J.; Luo, S.; Alzheimer's Disease Neuroimaging Initiative. Prediction of Conversion to Alzheimer's Disease with Longitudinal Measures and Time-To-Event Data. *J. Alzheimer's Dis.* 2017, *58*, 361–371. [CrossRef] [PubMed]
41. Xue, C.; Yuan, B.; Yue, Y.; Xu, J.; Wang, S.; Wu, M.; Ji, N.; Zhou, X.; Zhao, Y.; Rao, J.; et al. Distinct Disruptive Patterns of Default Mode Subnetwork Connectivity Across the Spectrum of Preclinical Alzheimer's Disease. *Front. Aging Neurosci.* 2019, *11*, 307. [CrossRef] [PubMed]
42. Li, C.; Yang, J.; Yin, X.; Liu, C.; Zhang, L.; Zhang, X.; Gui, L.; Wang, J. Abnormal intrinsic brain activity patterns in leukoaraiosis with and without cognitive impairment. *Behav. Brain Res.* 2015, *292*, 409–413. [CrossRef] [PubMed]

43. Frontzkowski, L.; Ewers, M.; Brendel, M.; Biel, D.; Ossenkoppele, R.; Hager, P.; Steward, A.; Dewenter, A.; Römer, S.; Rubinski, A.; et al. Earlier Alzheimer's disease onset is associated with tau pathology in brain hub regions and facilitated tau spreading. *Nat. Commun.* **2022**, *13*, 4899. [CrossRef] [PubMed]
44. King-Robson, J.; Wilson, H.; Politis, M.; Alzheimer's Disease Neuroimaging Initiative. Associations Between Amyloid and Tau Pathology, and Connectome Alterations, in Alzheimer's Disease and Mild Cognitive Impairment. *J. Alzheimer's Dis.* **2021**, *82*, 541–560. [CrossRef] [PubMed]

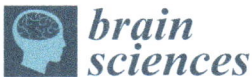

Article

Gross Total Resection Promotes Subsequent Recovery and Further Enhancement of Impaired Natural Killer Cell Activity in Glioblastoma Patients

Cheng-Chi Lee [1,2], Jeng-Fu You [2,3], Yu-Chi Wang [1,2], Shao-Wei Lan [1], Kuo-Chen Wei [1,2,4], Ko-Ting Chen [1,2], Yin-Cheng Huang [1,2], Tai-Wei Erich Wu [1] and Abel Po-Hao Huang [5,6,*]

1. Department of Neurosurgery, Chang Gung Memorial Hospital, Linkou, Taoyuan City 33305, Taiwan
2. College of Medicine, Chang Gung University, Taoyuan City 33302, Taiwan
3. Department of Colon and Rectal Surgery, Chang Gung Memorial Hospital, Linkou, Taoyuan City 33305, Taiwan
4. Department of Neurosurgery, New Taipei Municipal TuCheng Hospital, New Taipei City 236027, Taiwan
5. Institute of Polymer Science and Engineering, National Taiwan University, Taipei City 10663, Taiwan
6. Department of Surgery, College of Medicine, National Taiwan University Hospital, Taipei City 100229, Taiwan
* Correspondence: how.how0622@gmail.com

Highlights:

1. Natural killer cell activity is dramatically impaired in patients with glioblastoma.
2. Surgical resection of glioblastoma promotes redistribution of NK cell subsets and increases NK cell activity 30 days after surgery.
3. Gross total resection rather than subtotal resection significantly recovers and further increases the impaired NK cell activity in patients with glioblastoma.

Abstract: Glioblastoma is the most common primary malignant brain tumor, and median survival is relatively short despite aggressive standard treatment. Natural killer (NK) cell dysfunction is strongly associated with tumor recurrence and metastasis but is unclear in glioblastoma. NK activity (NKA) represents NK cell-secreted interferon-γ (IFN-γ), which modulates immunity and inhibits cancer progression. This study aimed to analyze NKA in glioblastoma patients to obtain a clearer overview of immunity surveillance. From 2020 to 2021, a total of 20 patients and six healthy controls were recruited. Peripheral blood samples were collected preoperatively and on postoperative days (POD) 3 and 30. Then, NKA was measured using the NK VUE kit. Although NKA decreased on POD3, it recovered and further significantly enhanced on POD30, with a nearly five-fold increase compared to baseline ($p = 0.004$). Furthermore, the percentage of $CD56^{bright}CD16^-$ NK cells decreased significantly on POD3 ($p = 0.022$) and further recovered on PO30. Subgroup analysis of extent surgical resection further revealed that the recovery of impaired NKA was attributable to gross total resection (GTR) rather than subtotal resection (STR). In conclusion, NKA is significantly impaired in glioblastoma, and GTR has demonstrated superior benefit in improving the suppressed NKA and increased $CD56^{bright}CD16^-$ NK subset in glioblastoma patients, which may be associated with subsequent patients' prognosis. Therefore, the goal of performing GTR for glioblastoma should be achieved when possible since it appears to increase NKA cell immunity.

Keywords: glioblastoma; natural killer cells; immune function; interferon; gross total resection

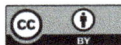

1. Introduction

Natural killer (NK) cells are granular lymphocytes of the innate immune system, and possess both innate and adaptive immune features [1,2]. Two main biological functions of NK cells for eliminating stressed, virus-infected, or malignant cells are direct NK cell-mediated cytotoxicity and indirect secretion of cytokines, such as interferon gamma (IFN-γ) [3–5]. In humans, NK cells are defined as $CD3^-CD56^+$ and/or $CD3^-CD16^+$ cells. In addition, NK cells can be further classified into two main subsets based on the expression level of CD16 and the cell surface density of CD56: the $CD56^{bright}CD16^-$ and $CD56^{dim}CD16^-$ NK cell subsets [6,7]. $CD56^{dim}CD16^+$ NK cells are the major circulating NK cell subset, comprising at least 90% of all peripheral blood NK cells, whereas approximately 10% of NK cells are $CD56^{bright}CD16^-$ subset [8]. $CD56^{bright}CD16^-$ NK cells have the capacity to secrete high amounts of cytokines such as IFN-γ but have less cytolytic activity. In contrast, $CD56^{dim}CD16^+$ NK cells possess significantly higher cytotoxic activity by producing much more perforin, granzymes and cytolytic granules. Although NK cell subsets can be determined based on their surface molecule repertoire under normal and different pathological conditions [9–11], the distribution of NK cell subsets in glioblastoma patients is still unclear.

Glioblastoma is the most common primary malignant brain tumor, accounting for 14.3% of all tumors and 49.1% of malignant central nervous system tumors [12,13]. The current standard of care for patients with glioblastoma is surgery, followed by a combination of radiation and chemotherapy. However, this aggressive therapeutic strategy has achieved only limited success, with a median overall survival (OS) of approximately 15 months and a median progression-free survival (PFS) of only approximately 6.2–7.5 months [14,15]. The dysfunction of immune cells, such as T cells and NK cells, has been recorded in association with physical trauma, such as thermal injury and surgery [16–19]. Moreover, evidence suggests that the immune dysfunction after surgery may be implicated in disease recurrence, metastasis and death [20]. It is still unknown, however, whether cranial surgery for glioblastoma affects the distribution of NK cell subtypes and their activity.

Many studies have demonstrated that NK cells are regarded as the major IFN-γ producer among peripheral blood mononuclear cells (PBMCs) for innate and adaptive immune responses [21,22]. NK cell-secreted IFN-γ is not only associated with cancer cell growth, apoptosis and tumor suppression, but is also correlates strongly with NK cell cytotoxicity [23–25]. In recent years, NK cell activity (NKA) has been widely measured by detecting secreted IFN-γ from NK cells in the ex vivo stimulated PBMC [26–28]. Therefore, the aim of this study was to investigate the influences of cranial surgical resection of glioblastoma on NKA and the distribution of NK cell subsets. Given the superior benefit of gross total resection (GTR) compared to subtotal resection (STR) in improving the survival outcomes [29,30], the impact of GTR or STR on NKA and NK cell subsets redistribution was also investigated.

2. Materials and Methods
2.1. Patients

This prospective study recruited 20 patients with histologically confirmed primary or recurrent glioblastoma treated in our institution between January 2020 and May 2021 and enrolled 6 healthy volunteers from our healthy center. The cancer types were determined according to the 2016 World Health Organization Classification of Tumors of the Central Nervous System [31]. Medical records of all participants were reviewed retrospectively, including tumor type, gender, age, and laboratory findings. The inclusion criteria for patients with glioblastoma in this study were (1) aged 20 or older; (2) patients with pathologically confirmed newly diagnosed or recurrent glioblastoma; and (3) receiving surgical resection of tumor. Patients with concomitant autoimmune disease, infectious, inflammatory process and/or with other second or occult tumors were excluded from this study. For healthy subjects, the inclusion criteria were (1) aged 20 years or older at the time of obtaining the informed consent; (2) medically healthy with no significant abnormal screening results clinically, such as vital signs, physical examination, electrocardiograms, and laboratory data; (3) no glioblastoma or other occult tumors; (4) no medical history of tumors; and (5) no previous or concurrent immune disease, infectious process or inflammatory state. Any subjects who did not fulfill the inclusion criteria were excluded.

2.2. Ethical Considerations and Surgical Resection of Glioblastoma

This study protocol was approved by the Institutional Review Board of Chang Gung Memorial Hospital (CGMH), Linkou, Taiwan (Number: 201900979B0) and conducted in accordance with the Helsinki Declaration. All included patients and healthy subjects provided signed informed consent to participate. The treatment decision for each patient was evaluated by a multidisciplinary team, including neurosurgeons, radiation oncologists, medical oncologists, neuroradiologists, and neuropathologists. Treatment decisions for each patient were evaluated by a multidisciplinary team including neuropathologists, neurooncologist, neurosurgeons, radiation oncologists, and medical oncologists. All patients underwent cranial surgical resection of glioblastoma. Surgical resection was performed to maximally remove the tumor mass and preserve as much functionally intact brain tissues as possible within the tumor boundaries. All patients received intravenous dexamethasone (Standard Chem & Pharm Co., Ltd., Tainan City, Taiwan) perioperatively (5 mg, q6h). The extent of resection was classified as GTR and STR based percentage of evaluable surgical removal, where GTR was defined as large than 95% resection, while STR was defined as 90–95% resection rate [32]. Peripheral blood samples were collected from glioblastoma patients preoperatively and on postoperative day (POD) 3 and 30.

2.3. Blood Sampling and Processing

Venous blood of patients and healthy controls was drawn into BD Vacutainer® Heparin Tubes coated with sodium heparin (BD Biosciences, Becton Dickinson, Franklin Lakes, NJ, USA). One milliliter of whole blood was transferred into NK VUE tube (NKMAX, Seongnam-si, Korea), and then the tube contents were gently mixed. After 20–24 h of incubation at 37 °C, the plasma was collected by centrifugation at $1200\times g$ for 4 min and stored at -20 °C. The remaining whole blood was used to isolate peripheral blood mononuclear cells (PBMCs) using Ficoll-Pague® (Cytiva, Marlborough, MA, USA) density gradient centrifugation. The isolated PBMCs were cryopreserved for later analysis.

2.4. Determination of NKA and Absolute NK Cell Counts

NKA was determined by measuring the secreted IFN-γ released by NK cells using the NK VUE Kit (NKMAX, Seongnam-si, Korea) according to the manufacturer's instructions. Briefly, cryopreserved plasma samples were thawed and centrifuged at $11,500\times g$ for 1 min at room temperature. Then, the supernatants were transferred into the diluent-loaded ELISA wells, and the mixtures were incubated for 1 h at room temperature. After washing away unbound material, IFN-γ was determined by anti-IFN-γ antibody conjugated to horseradish peroxidase (HRP). Subsequently, tetramethyl benzidine solution was aliquoted and incubated for 30 min following a wash to remove the unbound antibody-HRP complex. Finally, absorbance at 450 nm was measured and the amount of NK cell-secreted IFN-γ was quantitated. Absolute NK cell counts were determined from the peripheral blood of the patients and calculated using the formula WBC (cells/l) * Lymphocytes (%) * $CD3^-CD56^+$ and/or $CD3^-CD16^+$ cells (%).

2.5. Flow Cytometery Analysis

Cryopreserved PBMCs were thawed in a 37 °C water bath, and then transferred to a 15 mL centrifuge tube containing 5 mL of PBS. Then, PBMCs were incubated at 37 °C for 5 min, followed by centrifugation at $300\times g$ for 10 min. Next, the supernatants were discarded, and PBMCs were resuspended by adding 1 mL of PBS. After 1 h incubation at 37 °C, PBMCs were centrifuged at $300\times g$ for 10 min. Subsequently, PBMCs were resuspended and stained by the following monoclonal antibodies (mAbs) for 1 h: anti-CD3-PerCp-Cy5.5 (Catalog No. 560835), anti-CD4-APC (Catalog No. 555349), anti-CD8-FITC (Catalog No. 555366), anti-CD56-PE (Catalog No. 555516) and anti-CD16-BV421 (Catalog No. 562874). All mAbs were purchased from BD Biosciences (Becton Dickinson, Franklin Lakes, NJ, USA). Finally, stained PBMCs were analyzed using BD Fortessa flow cytometer (BD Biosciences, Becton Dickinson, Franklin Lakes, NJ, USA). Figure S1 shows the gating strategy for the analysis of NK cell and T cell phenotypes in single live lymphocytes by multiparametric flow cytometry.

2.6. Statistical Analysis

Statistical analyses were performed using SPSS software version 22 (IBM Corp., Armonk, NY, USA). Continuous data are presented as median with interquartile range, and categorical data are presented as frequency and percentage. The comparison between healthy controls and glioblastoma patients was statistically analyzed using a two-tailed Mann–Whitney U test. Intergroup comparisons were assessed with the Kruskal–Wallis test, followed by the two-tailed Wilcoxon matched-pairs signed-rank test. p values of less than 0.05 were considered statistically significant.

3. Results

3.1. Baseline Demographic and Clinical Characteristics of Patients with Glioblastoma

Table 1 shows the baseline demographic and clinical characteristics of glioblastoma patients. The median age of these patients was 61.5 years, ranging from 22 to 73 years (mean age: 58.4 ± 13.8 years). Most tumors were recurrent glioblastoma (75%) and located at frontal lobe (55%), parietal lobe (45%), and temporal lobe (20%). Diabetes (25%) was the most common comorbidity. Among them, 11 patients (55%) received gross total resection (GTR) and nine patients (45%) received subtotal resection (STR).

Table 1. Baseline demographic and clinical characteristics of glioblastoma patients (N = 20).

Variable	Glioblastoma Patients
Age, years, median (IQR)	61.5 (52.3–68.8)
Sex	
Male	9 (45.0%)
Female	11 (55.0%)
Glioblastoma	
Primary	5 (25.0%)
Recurrent	15 (75.0%)
Extent of resection	
GTR	11 (55.0%)
STR	9 (45.0%)
Tumor location	
Frontal lobe	11 (55.0%)
Parietal lobe	6 (30.0%)
Temporal lobe	4 (20.0%)
Insular	1 (5.0%)
Cerebellum	1 (5.0%)
Comorbidity	
Diabetes	5 (25.0%)
Dyslipidemia	3 (15.0%)
Hypertension	3 (15.0%)
Asthma	1 (5.0%)
Polyovarian syndrome	1 (5.0%)
CSDH	1 (5.0%)
Gout	1 (5.0%)
HBV Carrier	1 (5.0%)
Hepatitis C	1 (5.0%)
Thyroid goiters	1 (5.0%)
Time points of blood samples	
Baseline	20 (100%)
POD3	20 (100%)
POD30	14 (70.0%)

Continuous data are presented as median with interquartile range, and categorical data are presented as frequency and percentage. Abbreviations: GTR, gross total resection; CSDH, chronic subdural hematomas; HBV, hepatitis B virus; STR, subtotal resection; POD, postoperative days.

3.2. Impaired NKA Recovered 30 Days after Surgical Resection of Glioblastoma

In order to understand whether NKA is impaired in glioblastoma patients, we further recruited healthy subjects and compared the NKA status between glioblastoma patients and healthy control. As shown in Figure S2, glioblastoma patients had a significantly lower NKA than healthy subjects (21.8 pg/mL vs. 874.0 pg/mL, $p < 0.001$), suggesting that NKA is severely impaired in glioblastoma patients.

Next, we analyzed whether surgical resection of glioblastoma affects NKA status. Table 2 shows the NKA, NK count, and distribution of NK-cell and T-cell subsets in glioblastoma patients before surgical resection (baseline) and 3 days (POD3) and 30 days (POD30) after surgery. There were no statistically significant differences in the absolute NK counts and distribution of NK-cell and T-cell subsets between baseline, POD3, and POD30 ($p > 0.05$). However, NKA significantly differs between the baseline, POD3, and POD30 (21.8 pg/mL vs. 7.0 pg/mL vs. 107.6 pg/mL, $p = 0.001$). Figure 1A further shows the statistical analysis between baseline, POD3, and POD30. NKA was significantly decreased three days after surgical resection of glioblastoma (baseline vs. POD3, $p = 0.002$), but was significantly increased 30 days after surgery (baseline vs. POD30, $p = 0.002$). Notably, NKA at POD30 increased nearly five-fold compared with baseline (21.8 pg/mL vs. 107.6 pg/mL, $p = 0.004$), suggesting that surgical resection recovered the impaired NKA in glioblastoma patients. To clarify whether increased NKA after surgery was due to the increase of NK cell number, absolute NK cell counts from peripheral blood were analyzed. As shown in Figure 1B, there were no significant differences in absolute NK cell counts between baseline, POD3, and POD30 ($p > 0.05$).

Table 2. NKA status and distribution of NK cell and T cell subsets in patients with glioblastoma before and after surgical resection.

	Baseline	POD3	POD30	p-Value [†]
NKA (pg/mL)	21.8 (4.9, 76.5)	7.0 (1.9, 14.2)	107.6 (34.7, 457.9)	0.001
Absolute NK counts (cells/l)	160.99 (83.7, 325.36)	138.85 (62.39, 276.13)	192 (129.06, 262.89)	0.652
NK cell subset (n)				
CD56^{bright}CD16$^-$ NK cell (%)	1 (0.7, 3)	0.5 (0.3, 1.6)	0.7 (0.5, 1.2)	0.095
CD56^{dim}CD16$^+$ NK cell (%)	1 (0.7, 3)	0.5 (0.3, 1.6)	0.7 (0.5, 1.2)	0.095
T cell subset (n)				
CD4$^+$CD8$^-$ T cell (%)	41.3 (32.3, 57)	43.4 (29.8, 57.1)	39.5 (29.2, 68.6)	0.704
CD4$^-$CD8$^+$ T cell (%)	5.4 (3.1, 16.6)	7.5 (3.1, 16.8)	5.4 (2.6, 22.3)	0.382
CD56$^+$ T cell (%)	50 (30.7, 55.5)	46.2 (33.2, 59.4)	48.7 (26.7, 56.1)	0.342

Data are presented as median with IQR. [†] p-value was calculated using the Kruskal-Wallis H-test. Abbreviation: NKA, NK cell activity; NK cells, natural killer cells; POD, postoperative days; STR, subtotal resection; GTR, gross total resection.

3.3. Redistribution of NK Cell Subsets but Not T Cell Subsets after Cranial Surgery

Given the pleiotropic roles of different NK subsets on tumor immunity [33], we next examined whether surgical resection of glioblastoma affects the distribution of NK cell subsets as well as T cell subset. As shown in Figure 2A, the CD56^{bright}CD16$^-$ NK subset was significantly decreased on POD3 (median: 1.1% vs. 0.5%, $p = 0.022$, compared with baseline). Moreover, the CD56^{bright}CD16$^-$ NK subset was instead increased on POD30 (median: 0.5% vs. 0.7%, compared with POD3), although it did not reach statistical significance ($p > 0.05$). Conversely, CD56^{dim}CD16$^+$ NK subset was significantly increased on POD3 (median: 85.3% vs. 87.5%, $p = 0.04$, compared with baseline; Figure 2B), but further returned to baseline levels on POD30 (median: 85.3% vs. 84.7%, $p > 0.05$). On the other hand, the CD4$^+$CD8$^-$, CD4$^-$CD8$^+$, and CD56$^+$ T cell populations did not differ significantly between baseline, POD3, and POD30, suggesting that T cell subsets did not redistribute after surgery (All $p > 0.05$, Figure S3).

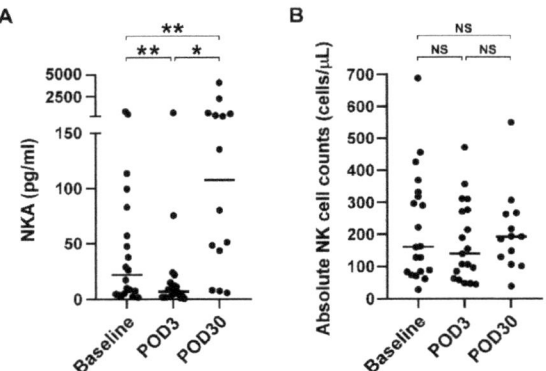

Figure 1. Impaired NKA recovered after surgical resection of glioblastoma on POD30. (**A**) NKA was measured before (baseline) and after surgical resection of glioblastoma on POD3 and POD30. NKA was determined by measuring the NK-released IFN-γ using the NK VUE kit. Data were presented as scatter plot, and differences between groups were statistically analyzed using the two-tailed Wilcoxon matched-pairs signed-rank test. Differences were found to be statistically significant at * $p < 0.05$ and ** $p < 0.01$. Solid line indicates the median. (**B**) Absolute NK cell counts were determined from patients before and after surgical resection of glioblastoma. Data were presented as scatter plot and median, and differences between groups were statistically analyzed using the two-tailed Wilcoxon matched-pairs signed-rank test. NS denotes no statistically significant difference. Abbreviation: NKA, natural killer cell activity; POD3, postoperative day 3; POD30, postoperative day 30.

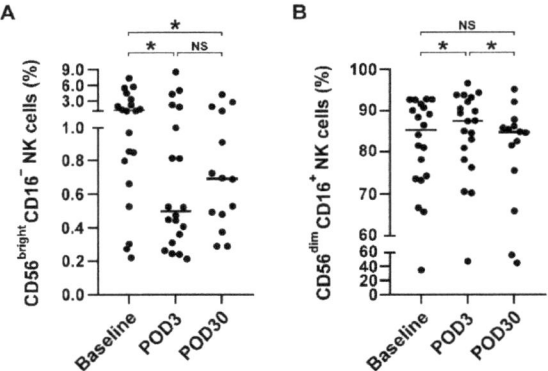

Figure 2. NK cell subsets were redistributed after cranial surgery. (**A**) Distribution of $CD56^{bright}CD16^-$ NK subsets before and after surgery. Surface expression of CD56 and CD16 were classified by flow cytometric analysis. (**B**) Distribution of $CD56^{dim}CD16^+$ NK subsets before and after surgery. Data were presented as scatter plot and median, and differences between groups were statistically analyzed using two-tailed Wilcoxon matched-pairs signed-rank test and. Differences were found to be statistically significant at * $p < 0.05$. NS indicates no statistically significant difference. Abbreviation: NK, natural killer; POD3, postoperative day 3; POD30, postoperative day 30.

3.4. NKA Is Significantly Increased on POD30 Compared with Baseline in Patients Receiving Gross Total Resection

Extent surgical resection is known to be independently associated with survival outcomes of patients with glioblastoma [34]. Therefore, we next investigated the impact of GTR or STR on NKA, absolute NK cell counts, and distribution of NK and T cell subsets. Table 3 shows the subgroup analysis of extent surgical resection using GTR and STR.

Regardless of GTR or STR subgroup, there were no significant differences in the absolute NK cell count and the distribution of NK- and T-cell subsets between baseline, POD3, and POD30 (all $p > 0.05$). However, NKA significantly differed between the baseline, POD3, and POD30 in glioblastoma patients who underwent GTR (7.7 vs. 5.0 vs. 153.5 pg/mL, $p = 0.001$). No significant differences were observed in NKA before and after STR (47.3 vs. 11.4 vs. 51.2 pg/mL, $p = 0.316$). Figure 3 further shows the statistical analysis between baseline, POD3 and POD30. There was no significant difference in NKA between patients before and 3 days after GTR (median: 7,7 vs. 5.0 pg/mL, $p = 0.155$, compared baseline with POD3). Notably, patients receiving GTR resulted in a substantial increase in NKA on POD30 (median: 7.7 vs. 153.5 pg/mL, $p = 0.015$, compared baseline with POD30). In contrast, NKA in patients who received STR was significantly decreased on POD3 (median: 47.3 vs. 11.4, $p = 0.008$, compared baseline with POD3), but returned to baseline on POD30 (median: 47.3 vs. 51.2 pg/mL, $p = 0.893$), suggesting that GTR rather than STR can recover the impaired NKA in patients with glioblastoma.

Table 3. NKA and NK cells in glioblastoma patients before and after GTR and STR.

	GTR (n = 11)				STR (n = 9)			
	Baseline	POD3	POD30	p-Value †	Baseline	POD3	POD30	p-Value †
NKA (pg/mL)	7.7 (3, 37.8)	5.0 (1.8, 11.2)	153.5 (45.9, 482.4)	0.001	47.3 (9.4, 250.2)	11.4 (2.5, 45.2)	51.2 (7.7, 1156.8)	0.316
Absolute NK count (cells/mL)	222.2 (83.2, 426.2)	105.7 (62.4, 270.7)	166.1 (117.4, 205.1)	0.619	160.3 (84.2, 296.5)	163.8 (77.3, 310.8)	262.9 (192.0, 266.4)	0.836
NK cell subset CD56^{bright}CD16$^-$ NK cell (%)	1.0 (0.5, 1.9)	0.5 (0.3, 1.8)	0.7 (0.6, 1.4)	0.260	1.4 (0.8, 3.9)	0.5 (0.4, 2.6)	0.4 (0.3, 1.6)	0.160
CD56^{dim}CD16$^+$ NK cell (%)	88.5 (74.2, 92.7)	89.4 (83, 93.3)	84.9 (82.0, 87.0)	0.478	80.9 (69.9, 90.4)	85.1 (73.2, 91.8)	75.4 (50.6, 89)	0.600
T cell subset CD4$^+$CD8$^-$ T cell (%)	42.8 (30.6, 72.5)	42.7 (22.9, 67.3)	39.8 (34.2, 69.3)	0.984	39.8 (33.9, 54.5)	44.1 (29.9, 52.1)	36.4 (29.2, 52.0)	0.956
CD4$^-$CD8$^+$ T cell (%)	47.7 (25.6, 54.5)	40.8 (30.1, 51.1)	46.8 (26.7, 55.7)	0.946	52.7 (36.2, 62.3)	50.6 (42, 60.7)	55.2 (43.2, 57.9)	0.998
CD56$^+$ T cell (%)	7.4 (3, 23.3)	8.2 (3.2, 19.4)	10.9 (4.6, 23.9)	0.886	3.5 (3.1, 10.3)	3.9 (2.2, 12.4)	2.6 (2.5, 3.5)	0.664

Abbreviation: GTR, gross total resection; STR, subtotal resection; NK, natural killer; NKA, natural killer cell activity; POD3, postoperative day 3; POD30, postoperative day 30. † p-value was calculated using Kruskal-Wallis test.

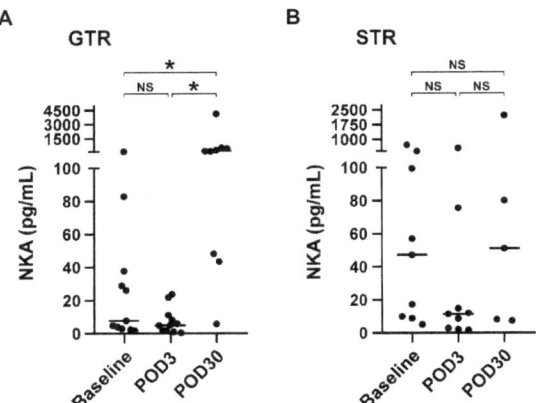

Figure 3. GTR rather than STR significantly recovered the impaired NKA at POD30. NKA of glioblastoma patients before (baseline) and after receiving GTR (**A**) or STR (**B**) on POD3 and POD30. Data were presented as scatter plot with median (solid line), and differences between groups were analyzed using two-tailed Mann-Whitney U test. * $p < 0.05$ was considered statistically significance between groups, while NS denotes no statistically significant difference. Abbreviation: NKA, NK cell activity; GTR, gross total resection; STR, subtotal resection; POD3, postoperative day 3; POD30, postoperative day 30.

4. Discussion

In this prospective study, we assessed NKA, NK cell counts, and the distribution of NK- and T-cell subsets in glioblastoma patients before and after surgery. Our results showed that glioblastoma patients have extremely low NKA compared with healthy subjects, indicating NK cell dysfunction in glioblastoma patients. Furthermore, surgical resection of glioblastoma not only redistributed NK cell subsets, but also greatly recovered the impaired NKA in glioblastoma patients 30 days after surgery. Stratified analysis further showed that the recovery of impaired NKA was attributable to GTR rather than STR. Therefore, the results of this study suggest that glioblastoma may have a negative impact on NK cell immunity, and that GTR is of great benefit in the recovery of impaired NKA in glioblastoma patients (Figure 4).

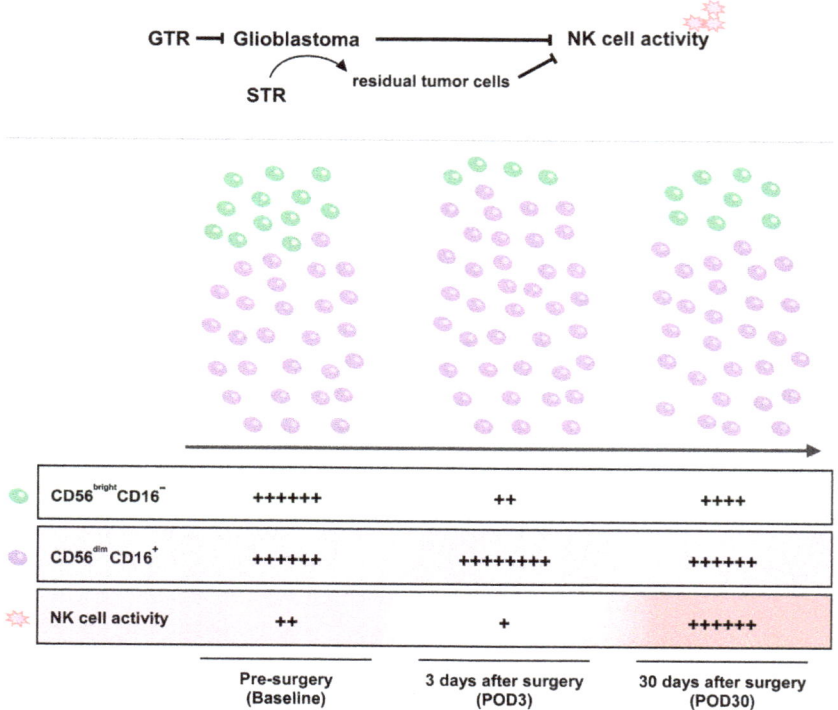

Figure 4. Schematic illustration of GTR in the recovery of the glioblastoma-suppressed natural killer cell activity with further enhancement.

Results of the present study found that NKA was further suppressed three days after cranial surgical resection of glioblastoma but recovered and further dramatically increased 30 days after surgery. Early postoperative NKA reduction is thought to be primarily attributable to the physiological response to surgical stress and a cascade of inflammatory responses, such as compensatory anti-inflammatory response [20,35]. Moreover, NK cell suppression after tumor surgery is considered to be a major driver of cancer metastasis and recurrence and is associated with poor survival outcomes [36]. In this study, early NK dysfunction after surgical resection of glioblastoma is also consistent with other studies of tumor resection. A study by Angka et al. [24] showed that NKA was dramatically reduced by 83.1% on POD1 in patients with colorectal cancer and gradually recovered after surgery. In a study of 24 pancreatic cancer patients, NK cell cytotoxicity was found to be significantly downregulated following pancreaticoduodenectomy on POD7 and return to baseline on POD30 [37]. Similar findings were also observed in Velasquez's study showing that NK function is significantly impaired after surgery for malignant bone tumors without significant changes in NK cell numbers [38]. It is worth noting that NKA in this study was significantly increased on POD30, even higher than baseline values, suggesting that a significant tumor burden had been resected, which may contribute to the gradual recovery of impaired NKA due to the suppression from glioblastoma. In addition, absolute NK cell numbers were not significantly different after surgery. Moreover, the recovery of impaired NKA was not due to an increase in NK cell numbers after surgery. Instead, it may be associated with changes in the redistribution of NK subsets or the quality of NK cells.

In this study, flow cytometric analysis was conducted to investigate whether impaired NKA stemmed from downregulation of CD56^{bright}CD16$^-$ NK cells, which is a subset of NK cells expressing the largest amount of IFN-γ. As expected, CD56^{bright}CD16$^-$ NK cells were significantly decreased on POD3, whereas CD56^{dim}CD16$^+$ NK cells were significantly increased. Although a previous study reported that CD56^{dim} NK cells also expressed IFN-γ within 4 h after triggering NK cell activation, CD56^{bright} NK cells produced the major IFN-γ after 16 h of stimulation [39]. Thus, we speculate that the major IFN-γ production in this study is from CD56^{bright} rather than CD56^{dim} NK cells. In other words, cranial surgery led to a redistribution of NK cell subsets from CD56^{bright}CD16$^-$ to CD56^{dim}CD16$^+$ within three days, which in turn lead to NKA downregulation. In addition to cell subset redistribution as a possible cause, the quality of NK cells may also have an impact on NKA. This is because that NKA dramatically increased nearly five-fold at POD30 compared with baseline, but the numbers of CD56^{bright}CD16$^-$ NK cells did not even return to baseline levels. Despite the current findings, more studies are needed to directly validate whether impaired NKA is due to redistribution and quality of NK cell subsets. On the other hand, several studies have demonstrated that T cells also express IFN- after specific stimulation [40–42]. Therefore, we further investigated whether surgical resection of glioblastoma could redistribute T cell subsets. Our data indicated that T cell subsets (CD4$^+$CD8$^-$, CD4$^-$CD8$^+$, CD56$^+$ T cell) were not affected after cranial surgery, i.e., T cells were not associated with NKA downregulation as a result of surgery.

In terms of potential therapeutics, steroids are often used in combination with cranial surgery, radiation therapy, and palliative care to reduce treatment-related toxicity [43]. Moreover, the use of steroid is known to suppress NK cell functions [44]. An immunophenotyping study by Chitadze et al. found that CD56^{bright} NK cells were significantly downregulated in glioblastoma patients treated with steroids, whereas steroid had no apparent impact on CD56^{dim} NK cells [45]. Vitale further indicated that the surface density of various activating NK receptors declined during methylprednisolone treatment, which is recognized as NK cell dysfunction, and then returned to normal levels shortly after steroid discontinuation or low-dose use [46]. Therefore, in this study, the decline of NKA and CD56^{bright} NK cells on POD3 after surgical removal glioblastoma may not be or slightly due to the steroid use. Nevertheless, in this study, the steroid was stopped about five days after the operation. This suggests that significant increase NKA and recovery of CD56^{bright} NK cells on POD30 may be mainly due to the evacuation of tumor cells, which eliminated the immune inhibition effect, and partly due to cessation of steroid usage.

In a recent comprehensive meta-analysis by Tang et al., GTR is superior to STR in terms of recurrence, survival rates, and functional outcomes in glioma patients [30]. It is generally believed that residual brain tumor cells closed to the resection border may remain alive and eventually reproliferate, leading to rapid recurrence. However, NK cells also play a key role in preventing tumor progression and metastasis through their direct cytotoxic activity and secreted cytokines [47]. Recent studies have shown that low NKA is significantly associated with a higher risk of various cancers, such as hepatocellular carcinoma [36], colorectal cancer [48], head and neck squamous cell carcinoma [49], lung cancer [50], and pancreatic cancer [51]. Jun's study showed that NKA is progressively impaired during tumor development, and its dysfunction is associated with recurrence and survival outcomes [52]. In this glioblastoma clinical study, we further found that glioblastoma was associated with lower NKA, and tumor resection facilitated NKA recovery, which was mainly attributable to GTR rather than STR. Importantly, during the recovery period after surgery, NKA rises, even above preoperative baseline levels, particularly in patients who received GTR. These results indicate that glioblastoma definitely had a negative impact on the immune system and that the goal of GTR should be achieved when it is possible in order to attain better immune rejuvenation and patient outcomes.

This study has several limitations, including the limited number of cases, which limits further identification of potential confounders associated with impaired NKA in glioblastoma and postoperative NKA recovery. The study was also conducted in a single institution and results may not be generalized to other populations. Some data were reviewed retrospectively from the medical records of prospectively included patients, which may preclude inferences of causality and may also limit long-term follow-up. Longer follow-up of NKA is necessary after completion of concurrent chemoradiation therapy and following treatment. In addition, although we recruited healthy volunteers to examine the NKA levels, incomplete demographic data of healthy subjects on variables may be considered a limitation of this study. Future prospective studies with a large sample size and healthy control are needed to further validate the finding of this study and improve the limitations associated with this study.

5. Conclusions

Glioblastoma progression has a great negative impact on the distribution of NK cell subtypes and their activity. NKA is significantly impaired in glioblastoma patients compared with healthy controls. During the recovery period after surgery, GTR rather than STR greatly restored the impaired NKA levels, even several folds higher than preoperative baseline levels. The unsatisfactory effect of STR may be due to continued inhibition of the activity of NK cells by residual tumor closed to the resection border. Therefore, the goal of performing GTR for glioblastoma should be achieved when possible since it appears to increase NK cell immunity. Further investigations are warranted to verify the role and function of these recovered NK cells after GTR in glioblastoma patients and to explore potential confounding factors affecting impaired NKA and GTR-dependent NKA recovery.

Supplementary Materials: The following supporting information can be downloaded at: https://www.mdpi.com/article/10.3390/brainsci12091144/s1, Figure S1: Gating strategy for identification of NK cell and T cell subsets. Figure S2: NKA was significantly downregulated in glioblastoma patients. Figure S3: T cell subsets were not redistributed before after cranial surgery.

Author Contributions: Conceptualization, C.-C.L. and A.P.-H.H.; resources, K.-C.W., C.-C.L., K.-T.C., J.-F.Y. and Y.-C.W.; formal analysis, S.-W.L. and T.-W.E.W.; writing—original draft preparation, C.-C.L., S.-W.L., J.-F.Y. and A.P.-H.H.; writing—review and editing, C.-C.L., Y.-C.W., Y.-C.H. and A.P.-H.H.; supervision, C.-C.L., K.-C.W. and Y.-C.H.; funding acquisition, C.-C.L., J.-F.Y. and K.-C.W. All authors have read and agreed to the published version of the manuscript.

Funding: This research was funded by Chang Gung Memorial Research Grand (Grant number: CMRPG1K0021).

Institutional Review Board Statement: The study was conducted according to the guidelines of the Declaration of Helsinki and approved by the Institutional Review Board of Chang Gung Memorial Hospital (CGMH), Linkou, Taiwan (Number: 201900979B0).

Informed Consent Statement: Informed consent was obtained from all subjects before participating in this study.

Acknowledgments: We acknowledged Chang Gung Memorial Hospital and University in support of this research.

Conflicts of Interest: The authors declare no conflict of interest.

References

1. Abel, A.M.; Yang, C.; Thakar, M.S.; Malarkannan, S. Natural Killer Cells: Development, Maturation, and Clinical Utilization. *Front. Immunol.* **2018**, *9*, 1869. [CrossRef]
2. Vivier, E.; Raulet, D.H.; Moretta, A.; Caligiuri, M.A.; Zitvogel, L.; Lanier, L.L.; Yokoyama, W.M.; Ugolini, S. Innate or adaptive immunity? The example of natural killer cells. *Science* **2011**, *331*, 44–49. [CrossRef]
3. Spits, H.; Artis, D.; Colonna, M.; Diefenbach, A.; Di Santo, J.P.; Eberl, G.; Koyasu, S.; Locksley, R.M.; McKenzie, A.N.; Mebius, R.E.; et al. Innate lymphoid cells—A proposal for uniform nomenclature. *Nat. Rev. Immunol.* **2013**, *13*, 145–149. [CrossRef]
4. Trinchieri, G.; Santoli, D.; Koprowski, H. Spontaneous cell-mediated cytotoxicity in humans: Role of interferon and immunoglobulins. *J. Immunol.* **1978**, *120*, 1849–1855.
5. Santoli, D.; Trinchieri, G.; Lief, F.S. Cell-mediated cytotoxicity against virus-infected target cells in humans. I. Characterization of the effector lymphocyte. *J. Immunol.* **1978**, *121*, 526–531.
6. Cooper, M.A.; Fehniger, T.A.; Caligiuri, M.A. The biology of human natural killer-cell subsets. *Trends Immunol.* **2001**, *22*, 633–640. [CrossRef]
7. Poli, A.; Michel, T.; Theresine, M.; Andres, E.; Hentges, F.; Zimmer, J. CD56bright natural killer (NK) cells: An important NK cell subset. *Immunology* **2009**, *126*, 458–465. [CrossRef]
8. Caligiuri, M.A. Human natural killer cells. *Blood* **2008**, *112*, 461–469. [CrossRef]
9. Freud, A.G.; Mundy-Bosse, B.L.; Yu, J.; Caligiuri, M.A. The Broad Spectrum of Human Natural Killer Cell Diversity. *Immunity* **2017**, *47*, 820–833. [CrossRef]
10. Melsen, J.E.; Lugthart, G.; Lankester, A.C.; Schilham, M.W. Human Circulating and Tissue-Resident CD56(bright) Natural Killer Cell Populations. *Front. Immunol.* **2016**, *7*, 262. [CrossRef]
11. Bjorkstrom, N.K.; Ljunggren, H.G.; Michaelsson, J. Emerging insights into natural killer cells in human peripheral tissues. *Nat. Rev. Immunol.* **2016**, *16*, 310–320. [CrossRef]
12. Low, J.T.; Ostrom, Q.T.; Cioffi, G.; Neff, C.; Waite, K.A.; Kruchko, C.; Barnholtz-Sloan, J.S. Primary brain and other central nervous system tumors in the United States (2014–2018): A summary of the CBTRUS statistical report for clinicians. *Neurooncol. Pract.* **2022**, *9*, 165–182. [CrossRef]
13. Ostrom, Q.T.; Cioffi, G.; Waite, K.; Kruchko, C.; Barnholtz-Sloan, J.S. CBTRUS Statistical Report: Primary Brain and Other Central Nervous System Tumors Diagnosed in the United States in 2014–2018. *Neuro Oncol.* **2021**, *23*, iii1–iii105. [CrossRef]
14. Marenco-Hillembrand, L.; Wijesekera, O.; Suarez-Meade, P.; Mampre, D.; Jackson, C.; Peterson, J.; Trifiletti, D.; Hammack, J.; Ortiz, K.; Lesser, E.; et al. Trends in glioblastoma: Outcomes over time and type of intervention: A systematic evidence based analysis. *J. Neurooncol.* **2020**, *147*, 297–307. [CrossRef]
15. Lakomy, R.; Kazda, T.; Selingerova, I.; Poprach, A.; Pospisil, P.; Belanova, R.; Fadrus, P.; Vybihal, V.; Smrcka, M.; Jancalek, R.; et al. Real-World Evidence in Glioblastoma: Stupp's Regimen After a Decade. *Front. Oncol.* **2020**, *10*, 840. [CrossRef]
16. Iversen, P.O.; Hjeltnes, N.; Holm, B.; Flatebo, T.; Strom-Gundersen, I.; Ronning, W.; Stanghelle, J.; Benestad, H.B. Depressed immunity and impaired proliferation of hematopoietic progenitor cells in patients with complete spinal cord injury. *Blood* **2000**, *96*, 2081–2083. [CrossRef]
17. Tai, L.H.; Zhang, J.; Scott, K.J.; de Souza, C.T.; Alkayyal, A.A.; Ananth, A.A.; Sahi, S.; Adair, R.A.; Mahmoud, A.B.; Sad, S.; et al. Perioperative influenza vaccination reduces postoperative metastatic disease by reversing surgery-induced dysfunction in natural killer cells. *Clin. Cancer Res.* **2013**, *19*, 5104–5115. [CrossRef]
18. Reinhardt, R.; Pohlmann, S.; Kleinertz, H.; Hepner-Schefczyk, M.; Paul, A.; Flohe, S.B. Invasive Surgery Impairs the Regulatory Function of Human CD56 bright Natural Killer Cells in Response to Staphylococcus aureus. Suppression of Interferon-gamma Synthesis. *PLoS ONE* **2015**, *10*, e0130155. [CrossRef]
19. Leaver, H.A.; Craig, S.R.; Yap, P.L.; Walker, W.S. Lymphocyte responses following open and minimally invasive thoracic surgery. *Eur. J. Clin. Investig.* **2000**, *30*, 230–238. [CrossRef]
20. Market, M.; Tennakoon, G.; Auer, R.C. Postoperative Natural Killer Cell Dysfunction: The Prime Suspect in the Case of Metastasis Following Curative Cancer Surgery. *Int. J. Mol. Sci.* **2021**, *22*, 11378. [CrossRef]
21. Pellegatta, S.; Eoli, M.; Frigerio, S.; Antozzi, C.; Bruzzone, M.G.; Cantini, G.; Nava, S.; Anghileri, E.; Cuppini, L.; Cuccarini, V.; et al. The natural killer cell response and tumor debulking are associated with prolonged survival in recurrent glioblastoma patients receiving dendritic cells loaded with autologous tumor lysates. *Oncoimmunology* **2013**, *2*, e23401. [CrossRef]
22. Paul, S.; Lal, G. The Molecular Mechanism of Natural Killer Cells Function and Its Importance in Cancer Immunotherapy. *Front. Immunol.* **2017**, *8*, 1124. [CrossRef]
23. Cui, F.; Qu, D.; Sun, R.; Zhang, M.; Nan, K. NK cell-produced IFN-gamma regulates cell growth and apoptosis of colorectal cancer by regulating IL-15. *Exp. Ther. Med.* **2020**, *19*, 1400–1406. [CrossRef]
24. Angka, L.; Martel, A.B.; Kilgour, M.; Jeong, A.; Sadiq, M.; de Souza, C.T.; Baker, L.; Kennedy, M.A.; Kekre, N.; Auer, R.C. Natural Killer Cell IFNgamma Secretion is Profoundly Suppressed Following Colorectal Cancer Surgery. *Ann. Surg. Oncol.* **2018**, *25*, 3747–3754. [CrossRef]
25. Perera Molligoda Arachchige, A.S. Human NK cells: From development to effector functions. *Innate Immun.* **2021**, *27*, 212–229. [CrossRef]

26. Lee, S.B.; Cha, J.; Kim, I.K.; Yoon, J.C.; Lee, H.J.; Park, S.W.; Cho, S.; Youn, D.Y.; Lee, H.; Lee, C.H.; et al. A high-throughput assay of NK cell activity in whole blood and its clinical application. *Biochem. Biophys. Res. Commun.* **2014**, *445*, 584–590. [CrossRef]
27. Lee, Y.K.; Haam, J.H.; Suh, E.; Cho, S.H.; Kim, Y.S. A Case-Control Study on the Changes in Natural Killer Cell Activity following Administration of Polyvalent Mechanical Bacterial Lysate in Korean Adults with Recurrent Respiratory Tract Infection. *J. Clin. Med.* **2022**, *11*, 3014. [CrossRef]

28. Jung, Y.S.; Park, J.H.; Park, D.I.; Sohn, C.I.; Lee, J.M.; Kim, T.I. Impact of Smoking on Human Natural Killer Cell Activity: A Large Cohort Study. *J. Cancer Prev.* **2020**, *25*, 13–20. [CrossRef]
29. Han, Q.; Liang, H.; Cheng, P.; Yang, H.; Zhao, P. Gross Total vs. Subtotal Resection on Survival Outcomes in Elderly Patients With High-Grade Glioma: A Systematic Review and Meta-Analysis. *Front. Oncol.* **2020**, *10*, 151. [CrossRef]
30. Tang, S.; Liao, J.; Long, Y. Comparative assessment of the efficacy of gross total versus subtotal total resection in patients with glioma: A meta-analysis. *Int. J. Surg.* **2019**, *63*, 90–97. [CrossRef]
31. Louis, D.N.; Perry, A.; Reifenberger, G.; von Deimling, A.; Figarella-Branger, D.; Cavenee, W.K.; Ohgaki, H.; Wiestler, O.D.; Kleihues, P.; Ellison, D.W. The 2016 World Health Organization Classification of Tumors of the Central Nervous System: A summary. *Acta Neuropathol.* **2016**, *131*, 803–820. [CrossRef]
32. Ahmed, F.I.; Abdullah, K.G.; Durgin, J.; Salinas, R.D.; O'Rourke, D.M.; Brem, S. Evaluating the Association Between the Extent of Resection and Survival in Gliosarcoma. *Cureus* **2019**, *11*, e4374. [CrossRef]
33. Corvino, D.; Kumar, A.; Bald, T. Plasticity of NK cells in Cancer. *Front. Immunol.* **2022**, *13*, 888313. [CrossRef]
34. Wang, L.; Liang, B.; Li, Y.I.; Liu, X.; Huang, J.; Li, Y.M. What is the advance of extent of resection in glioblastoma surgical treatment-a systematic review. *Chin. Neurosurg. J.* **2019**, *5*, 2. [CrossRef]
35. Angka, L.; Khan, S.T.; Kilgour, M.K.; Xu, R.; Kennedy, M.A.; Auer, R.C. Dysfunctional Natural Killer Cells in the Aftermath of Cancer Surgery. *Int. J. Mol. Sci.* **2017**, *18*, 1787. [CrossRef]
36. Lee, H.A.; Goh, H.G.; Lee, Y.S.; Jung, Y.K.; Kim, J.H.; Yim, H.J.; Lee, M.G.; An, H.; Jeen, Y.T.; Yeon, J.E.; et al. Natural killer cell activity is a risk factor for the recurrence risk after curative treatment of hepatocellular carcinoma. *BMC Gastroenterol.* **2021**, *21*, 258. [CrossRef] [PubMed]
37. Iannone, F.; Porzia, A.; Peruzzi, G.; Birarelli, P.; Milana, B.; Sacco, L.; Dinatale, G.; Peparini, N.; Prezioso, G.; Battella, S.; et al. Effect of surgery on pancreatic tumor-dependent lymphocyte asset: Modulation of natural killer cell frequency and cytotoxic function. *Pancreas* **2015**, *44*, 386–393. [CrossRef]
38. Velasquez, J.F.; Ramirez, M.F.; Ai, D.I.; Lewis, V.; Cata, J.P. Impaired Immune Function in Patients Undergoing Surgery for Bone Cancer. *Anticancer Res.* **2015**, *35*, 5461–5466.
39. De Maria, A.; Bozzano, F.; Cantoni, C.; Moretta, L. Revisiting human natural killer cell subset function revealed cytolytic CD56(dim)CD16+ NK cells as rapid producers of abundant IFN-gamma on activation. *Proc. Natl. Acad. Sci. USA* **2011**, *108*, 728–732. [CrossRef]
40. Verhoef, C.M.; Van Roon, J.A.; Vianen, M.E.; Glaudemans, C.A.; Lafeber, F.P.; Bijlsma, J.W. Lymphocyte stimulation by CD3-CD28 enables detection of low T cell interferon-gamma and interleukin-4 production in rheumatoid arthritis. *Scand. J. Immunol.* **1999**, *50*, 427–432. [CrossRef]
41. Benvenuto, F.; Voci, A.; Carminati, E.; Gualandi, F.; Mancardi, G.; Uccelli, A.; Vergani, L. Human mesenchymal stem cells target adhesion molecules and receptors involved in T cell extravasation. *Stem. Cell Res. Ther.* **2015**, *6*, 245. [CrossRef] [PubMed]
42. Yu, S.F.; Zhang, Y.N.; Yang, B.Y.; Wu, C.Y. Human memory, but not naive, CD4+ T cells expressing transcription factor T-bet might drive rapid cytokine production. *J. Biol. Chem.* **2014**, *289*, 35561–35569. [CrossRef] [PubMed]
43. Ryken, T.C.; Kuo, J.S.; Prabhu, R.S.; Sherman, J.H.; Kalkanis, S.N.; Olson, J.J. Congress of Neurological Surgeons Systematic Review and Evidence-Based Guidelines on the Role of Steroids in the Treatment of Adults With Metastatic Brain Tumors. *Neurosurgery* **2019**, *84*, E189–E191. [CrossRef]
44. Capellino, S.; Claus, M.; Watzl, C. Regulation of natural killer cell activity by glucocorticoids, serotonin, dopamine, and epinephrine. *Cell Mol. Immunol.* **2020**, *17*, 705–711. [CrossRef]
45. Chitadze, G.; Fluh, C.; Quabius, E.S.; Freitag-Wolf, S.; Peters, C.; Lettau, M.; Bhat, J.; Wesch, D.; Oberg, H.H.; Luecke, S.; et al. In-depth immunophenotyping of patients with glioblastoma multiforme: Impact of steroid treatment. *Oncoimmunology* **2017**, *6*, e1358839. [CrossRef]
46. Vitale, C.; Chiossone, L.; Cantoni, C.; Morreale, G.; Cottalasso, F.; Moretti, S.; Pistorio, A.; Haupt, R.; Lanino, E.; Dini, G.; et al. The corticosteroid-induced inhibitory effect on NK cell function reflects down-regulation and/or dysfunction of triggering receptors involved in natural cytotoxicity. *Eur. J. Immunol.* **2004**, *34*, 3028–3038. [CrossRef]
47. Bassani, B.; Baci, D.; Gallazzi, M.; Poggi, A.; Bruno, A.; Mortara, L. Natural Killer Cells as Key Players of Tumor Progression and Angiogenesis: Old and Novel Tools to Divert Their Pro-Tumor Activities into Potent Anti-Tumor Effects. *Cancers* **2019**, *11*, 461. [CrossRef]
48. Furue, H.; Matsuo, K.; Kumimoto, H.; Hiraki, A.; Suzuki, T.; Yatabe, Y.; Komori, K.; Kanemitsu, Y.; Hirai, T.; Kato, T.; et al. Decreased risk of colorectal cancer with the high natural killer cell activity NKG2D genotype in Japanese. *Carcinogenesis* **2008**, *29*, 316–320. [CrossRef]
49. Charap, A.J.; Enokida, T.; Brody, R.; Sfakianos, J.; Miles, B.; Bhardwaj, N.; Horowitz, A. Landscape of natural killer cell activity in head and neck squamous cell carcinoma. *J. Immunother. Cancer* **2020**, *8*, e001623. [CrossRef]
50. Borg, M.; Wen, S.W.C.; Hansen, T.F.; Jakobsen, A.; Andersen, R.F.; Hilberg, O.; Weinreich, U.M.; Nederby, L. Natural killer cell activity as a biomarker for the diagnosis of lung cancer in high-risk patients. *J. Int. Med. Res.* **2022**, *50*, 3000605221108924. [CrossRef]

51. Marcon, F.; Zuo, J.; Pearce, H.; Nicol, S.; Margielewska-Davies, S.; Farhat, M.; Mahon, B.; Middleton, G.; Brown, R.; Roberts, K.J.; et al. NK cells in pancreatic cancer demonstrate impaired cytotoxicity and a regulatory IL-10 phenotype. *Oncoimmunology* **2020**, *9*, 1845424. [CrossRef] [PubMed]
52. Jun, E.; Song, A.Y.; Choi, J.W.; Lee, H.H.; Kim, M.Y.; Ko, D.H.; Kang, H.J.; Kim, S.W.; Bryceson, Y.; Kim, S.C.; et al. Progressive Impairment of NK Cell Cytotoxic Degranulation Is Associated With TGF-beta1 Deregulation and Disease Progression in Pancreatic Cancer. *Front. Immunol.* **2019**, *10*, 1354. [CrossRef] [PubMed]

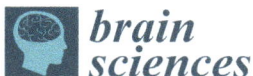

Article

Endovascular Treatment of ICAS Patients: Targeting Reperfusion Rather than Residual Stenosis

Tingyu Yi [1], Alai Zhan [2], Yanmin Wu [1], Yimin Li [2], Xiufen Zheng [1], Dinglai Lin [1], Xiaohui Lin [1], Zhinan Pan [1], Rongcheng Chen [1], Mark Parsons [3], Wenhuo Chen [1,*] and Longting Lin [3,*]

1. Cerebrovascular and Neuro-Intervention Department, Zhangzhou Affiliated Hospital of Fujian Medical University, Zhangzhou 363000, China; siyuyufen@163.com (T.Y.); minmindoc@163.com (Y.W.); zxf5860@163.com (X.Z.); lindinglai1@163.com (D.L.); linxh@foxmail.com (X.L.); m18050700089@163.com (Z.P.); crc337617@163.com (R.C.)
2. Radiology Department, Zhangzhou Affiliated Hospital of Fujian Medical University, Zhangzhou 363000, China; zhanalai@163.com (A.Z.); bluecorn324115@163.com (Y.L.)
3. Department of Neurology and Medicine, Royal Melbourne Hospital, University of Melbourne, Melbourne, VIC 3050, Australia; mark.parsons@unsw.edu.au
* Correspondence: doctorwwenhuo@126.com (W.C.); longting.lin@uon.edu.au (L.L.); Tel.: +86-13806906089 (W.C.); +86-13777446074 (L.L.)

Abstract: Background and Purpose: Previous studies showed that acute reocclusion after endovascular therapy is related to residual stenosis. However, we observed that reperfusion status but not residual stenosis severity is related to acute reocclusion. This study aimed to assess which factor mention above is more likely to be associated with artery reocclusion after endovascular treatment. Methods: This study included 86 acute ischemic stroke patients who had middle cerebral artery (MCA) atherosclerotic occlusions and received endovascular treatment within 24 h of a stroke. The primary outcomes included intraprocedural reocclusion assessed during endovascular treatment and delayed reocclusion assessed through follow-up angiography. Results: Of the 86 patients, the intraprocedural reocclusion rate was 7.0% (6/86) and the delayed reocclusion rate was 2.3% (2/86). Regarding intraprocedural occlusion, for patients with severe residual stenosis, patients with successful thrombectomy reperfusion showed a significantly lower rate than unsuccessful thrombectomy reperfusion (0/30 vs. 6/31, $p = 0.003$); on the other hand, for patients with successful thrombectomy reperfusion, patients with severe residual stenosis showed no difference from those with mild to moderate residual stenosis in terms of intraprocedural occlusion (0/30 vs. 0/25, $p = 1.00$). In addition, after endovascular treatment, all patients achieved successful reperfusion. There was no significant difference in the delayed reocclusion rate between patients with severe residual stenosis and those with mild to moderate residual stenosis (2/25 vs. 0/61, $p = 0.085$). Conclusion: Reperfusion status rather than residual stenosis severity is associated with artery reocclusion after endovascular treatment. Once successful reperfusion was achieved, the reocclusion occurrence was fairly low in MCA atherosclerosis stroke patients, even with severe residual stenosis.

Keywords: atherosclerotic; residual stenosis; reocclusion; endovascular treatment

1. Introduction

Endovascular therapy (EVT) has become a routine practice for acute ischemic stroke caused by large vessel occlusion in highly specialized centers with dedicated stroke units [1,2]. However, EVT procedures do not always lead to good clinical outcomes. One of the reasons is reocclusion of the targeted artery after procedure. The incidence of postoperative acute reocclusion of treated arteries has been reported to range from 3 to 9% [3], and the incidence has been shown to be higher in cases of intracranial atherosclerosis (ICAS)-related occlusion, especially in cases with high residual stenosis [4], because insufficient blood flow caused by high residual stenosis through the target artery leads to acute thrombus formation [4–6]. Therefore, if there is sufficient blood flow through the occluded artery affected by ICAS, the incidence of acute thrombosis after endovascular therapy can be relatively low. Furthermore, in our clinical practice, we observed that unsuccessful reperfusion as defined by mTICI < 2b rather than residual stenosis severity was related to artery reocclusion in ICAS patients. We hypothesized that the incidence of acute target arterial reocclusion would be low if mTICI $\geq$ 2b reperfusion was achieved in patients with MCA ICAS-related occlusion even with high degree of residual stenosis after endovascular therapy. Therefore, our study aimed to assess whether reocclusion was determined by reperfusion status or residual stenosis severity in ICAS patients.

2. Methods

2.1. Study Design

This retrospective study included the following two-step analysis: (1) Step 1: intraprocedural reocclusion analysis during EVT; (2) Step 2: delayed reocclusion analysis through follow-up angiographic images. Intraprocedural reocclusion was defined as reocclusion during the EVT procedure. Delayed reocclusion was assessed by examining follow-up (2–7 days) angiographic images, which was defined as a sudden cutoff without a distal flow in magnetic resonance angiography or without the presence of distal flow in computed topography angiography. Reocclusion were evaluated by 2 independent raters (Z.A.L. and L.Y.M).

For Step 1 (analysis of intraprocedural reocclusion), the patients were divided into 3 groups based on the angiographic results during the thrombectomy procedure: Group 1a: successful thrombectomy reperfusion (TICI 2b or 3) + mild to moderate stenosis; Group 2a: successful thrombectomy reperfusion + severe stenosis; and Group 3a: no successful thrombectomy reperfusion + severe stenosis. For Step 2 (analysis of delayed reocclusion), the patients were divided into two groups based on the final angiographic result at the end of the EVT: Group 1b: successful reperfusion + mild-to-moderate stenosis; Group 2b: successful reperfusion + severe stenosis.

2.2. Patients

From our prospective registry database, acute ischemic stroke patients admitted between January 2015 and July 2019 were retrospectively reviewed. Patients with anterior circulation stroke and who received EVT within 24 h of stroke onset were selected. Further inclusion criteria were as follows: (1) middle cerebral artery occlusion (tandem occlusion was not included); (2) a diagnosis of ICAS; (3) successful reperfusion that was characterized by a modified thrombolysis in cerebral ischemia (mTICI) Grade 2b to 3 at the end of EVT. Patients with arterial fibrillation that could easily cause cardiac embolism [7] were excluded from this study. Further exclusion criteria were as follows: (1) partial baseline occlusion, (2) no follow-up imaging, and (3) poor imaging quality. The study was approved by the institution's ethical committee.

2.3. Endovascular Procedures

Thrombectomy with stent retrieval was the first endovascular strategy, with emergent angioplasty and/or a stent as a rescue treatment after 1–2 passes of thrombectomy. If successful thrombectomy reperfusion was achieved and could be maintained for more than 20 min, the endovascular therapy was terminated.

2.4. Tirofiban Administration and Antiplatelet Regime

A loading dose (10 µg/kg) of a glycoprotein IIb/IIIa inhibitor (tirofiban) was administered intravenously for 3 min once ICAS was considered as the cause of the stroke during the EVT procedure (prior to attempting thrombectomy), then an infusion of tirofiban at 0.1–0.15 µg/kg/min was administered, and this infusion was continued for 12–36 h after the EVT operation [8]. If no brain hemorrhages were detected by the CT scan performed at least 12 h after the operation, a loading dose of aspirin (100 mg/day) plus clopidogrel

(300 mg/day), followed by a dose of aspirin (100 mg/day) plus clopidogrel (75 mg/day) for at least 3 months was administered to both patients who received stenting and those who did not.

2.5. Definitions of ICAS

ICAS was suspected once the following signs were observed on the first run of DSA: the appearance of a tapered sign [9] or/and significant fixed focal stenosis (>50%) at the site of occlusion during endovascular treatment [10] or/and the phenomenon of "microcrater first-pass effect" [11], or/and a positive stent-unsheathed effect [12]. In addition, a subgroup of patients was scanned by follow-up high-resolution magnetic resonance imaging to confirm the definition.

2.6. Evaluation of Angiographic Images

All angiographic classifications, including the grade of collateral flow, the degree of residual stenosis, and the reperfusion score, were evaluated by the two independent raters who rated the reocclusion status (Z.A.L. and L.Y.M). Interobserver disagreements were resolved by consensus.

The baseline grade of collateral flow was evaluated according to the American Society of Interventional and Therapeutic Neuroradiology/Society of Interventional Radiology Collateral Flow Grading System (ASTRIN) through pretreatment angiography. According to this angiographic scale, collateral flow can be classified into Grades 0 to 4 according to the completeness and rapidity of collateral filling in a retrograde manner [13].

The reperfusion statuses was measured using the Thrombolysis in Cerebral Infarction (TICI) scale [13]. An mTICI of 2b-3 was classified as successful reperfusion.

The degree of stenosis was measured by the Warfarin–Aspirin Symptomatic Intracranial Disease Study (WASID) method. The degree of stenosis was classified as mild to moderate (<70%) or high (70–99%) [14].

2.7. Outcomes

The primary outcome for Step 1 of the analysis was intraprocedural reocclusion. The primary outcome for Step 2 of the analysis was delayed reocclusion. The secondary outcomes included 3-month favorable outcome defined by a modified Rankin score (mRS) of 0–2, and symptomatic intracranial hemorrhage (sICH), defined as any type of hemorrhage associated with an increase in the National Institutes of Health Stroke Scale (NIHSS) score by ≥ 4 points within 72 h.

2.8. Statistical Analysis

Statistical analysis was performed using the SPSS statistical package (version 20.0, Chicago, IL, USA). For the comparison between two groups, a χ^2 test was performed for categorical variables, Student's *t*-test was performed for continuous variables with a normal distribution, and Mann–Whitney's U-test was performed for continuous variables without a normal distribution or ordinal variables. ANOVA was performed for the comparison among three groups, followed by Bonferroni correction for pairwise comparison.

3. Results

3.1. Patients

This study included 855 acute anterior circulation stroke patients, of whom 394 had an occlusion on the middle cerebral artery. Of the 394 patients, 107 were included with a diagnosis of ICAS, and 103 out of the 107 patients were further included with successful reperfusion after EVT. Next, 17 out of the 103 patients were excluded due to partial baseline occlusion (N = 12), no follow-up imaging (N = 3), or poor imaging quality (N = 2). Therefore, a total of 86 patients were selected for the study. All patients received tirofiban treatment. No patients received endarterectomy, which is one treatment for carotid artery stenosis [15] in this cohort. The patient selection process is detailed in Figure 1 and a detailed decision-making flow chart is depicted in Figure 2.

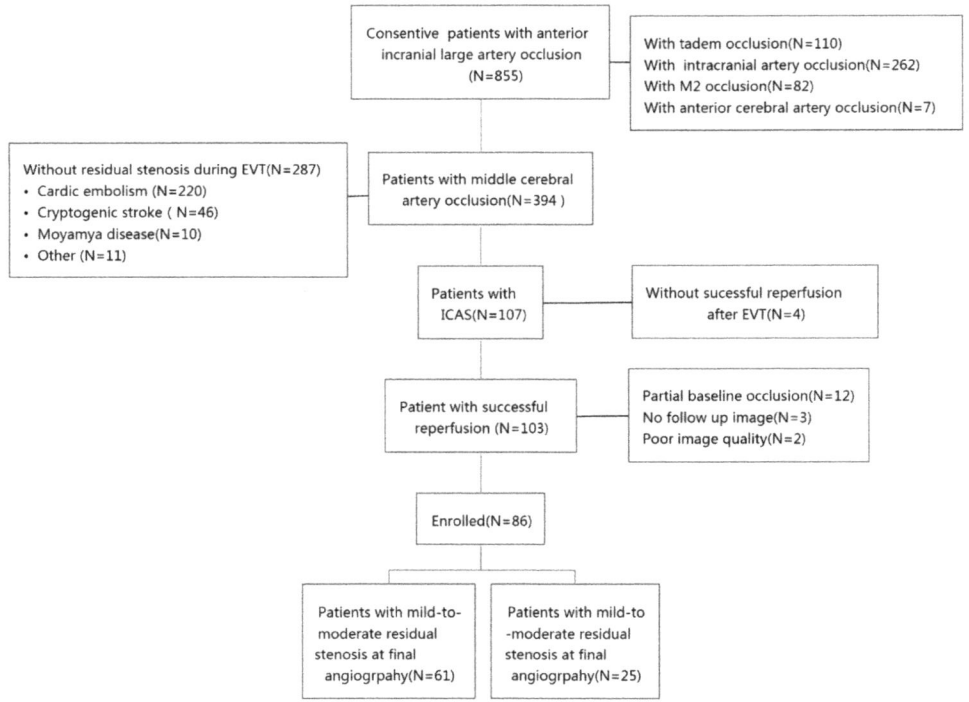

Figure 1. Patient selection and exclusion flow chart.

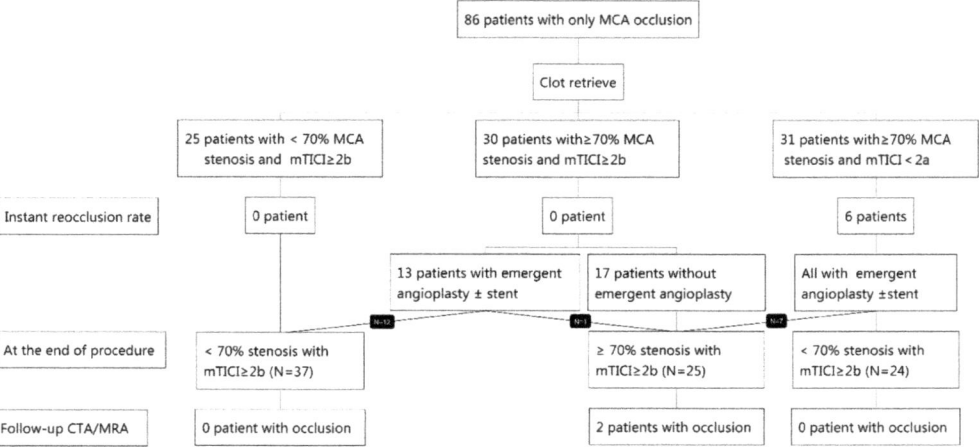

Figure 2. Decision-making flow chart. EVT, endovascular therapy; MCA, middle cerebral artery; mTICI, modified thrombolysis in cerebral infarction; CTA, computed tomography angiography; MRA, magnetic resonance angiography.

3.2. ICAS Classification Validation

Twenty-two patients underwent high-resolution magnetic resonance imaging, and acentric plaques could be observed in all these cases, which confirmed the diagnosis of ICAS.

3.2.1. Step 1 Analysis: Intraprocedural Reocclusion

The intraprocedural reocclusion rate of the whole cohort was 7.0% (6/86), with a significant difference among the three groups (p = 0.003, Table 1). Pairwise comparison showed that for the patients with successful thrombectomy reperfusion, those with severe residual stenosis showed no difference from those with mild to moderate residual stenosis in terms of the intraprocedural reocclusion rate (Group 2a vs. Group 1a, 0/30 vs. 0/25, p = 1.0); on the other hand, for patients with severe residual stenosis, those with successful thrombectomy reperfusion showed a significantly lower intraprocedural reocclusion rate compared with no successful thrombectomy reperfusion (Group 2a vs. Group 3a, 0/30 vs. 6/31, p = 0.007).

Table 1. Baseline characteristics and clinical outcomes of patients in Step 1 of the analysis.

	Group 1a: mTICI $\geq$ 2b + Stenosis < 70% (N = 25)	Group 2a: mTICI $\geq$ 2b + Stenosis $\geq$ 70% (N = 30)	Group 3a: mTICI < 2b + Stenosis $\geq$ 70% (N = 31)	p-Value
Male Sex, N (%)	18 (72%)	22 (73.3%)	22 (71.0%)	0.979
Age (mean, years)	64 ± 15	66 ± 10	62 ± 12	0.497
Smoker	10 (40%)	16 (51.6%)	17 (56.7%)	0.457
Hypertension, N (%)	16 (72.7%)	24 (80.0%)	26 (86.7%)	0.454
DM N (%)	7 (28.0%)	8 (26.7%)	9 (29.0%)	0.979
Atrial fibrillation N (%)	0 (0%)	1 (3.3%)	0 (0%)	0.389
TIA N (%)	1 (4.0%)	1 (3.3%)	0 (0%)	0.554
Admission NIHSS (median, IQR)	14 (11,18)	13 (11,17)	14 (11,18)	0.332
Onset-to-puncture time N (%)				0.022
Within 8 h	18 (72%)	20 (66.7%)	12 (38.7%)	
8–24 h	7 (28%)	10 (33.3%)	19 (61.3%)	
Good collateral flow, N (%)				
ASITN $\geq$ 3	14 (56.0%)	24 (77.4%)	15 (50.0%)	0.070
Instant reocclusion	0 (0%)	0 (0%)	6 (19.4%)	0.03

mTICI, modified thrombolysis in cerebral infarction; TIA, transient ischemic attack; DM, diabetes mellitus; NIHSS, National Institutes of Health Stroke Scale; IQR, interquartile range; ASITN, American Society of Interventional and Therapeutic Neuroradiology collateral grading system.

The clinical and angiography characteristics of the three groups are summarized in Table 1. The baseline characteristics were similar among the three groups except for onset-to-groin puncture time. Group 3a (patients with severe residual stenosis but successful thrombectomy reperfusion) had more patients receiving thrombectomy beyond 8 h of onset compared with the other two groups (61.3% vs. 33.3% vs. 28%, p = 0.022).

3.2.2. Step 2 Analysis: Delayed Occlusion

Moreover, for the group of patients with no successful thrombectomy reperfusion (N = 31, Group 3a from Step 1), the intraprocedural reocclusion rate was 19.4% (6/31); however, after successful reperfusion with the rescue treatment, this group of patients had a lower intraprocedural reocclusion rate (0/31 vs. 6/31, p = 0.032).

At the end of the EVT procedure, after rescue treatment of angioplasty and/or a stent, all patients achieved successful reperfusion after the EVT procedure. For the whole cohort, the delayed reocclusion rate was 2.3% (2/86), the rate of sICH was 1.2% (1/86), and the rate of good prognosis was 66.3% (57/86).

Sixty-one patients had mild to moderate residual stenosis (Group 1b), whereas 25 patients had severe residual stenosis (Group 2b, a typical case is illustrated in Figure 3). The two groups showed no significant difference regarding the reocclusion rate on follow-up angioplasty (0/61 vs. 2/25, p = 0.082). The two groups showed no significant difference in sICH (0/61 vs. 1/25, p = 0.298) or favorable functional outcome prognosis rate (41/61 vs.

16/25, p = 0.808, Table 2). The clinical and angiography characteristics of the three groups are summarized in Table 2.

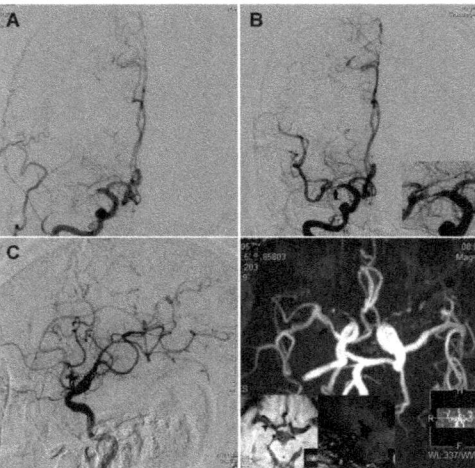

Figure 3. An ICAS case with a high degree of residual stenosis. An elderly patient presented with left limb weakness for 16 h, and the NIHSS score was 14. (**A**) The first run of DSA showed occlusion of the right MCA. (**B**) The anterior–posterior view of DSA showed a high degree of stenosis (black arrow) located at the right MCA after one pass of stent retrieval and emergent angioplasty via a 2.0–15 mm Maverick balloon; as the figure on the bottom right shows, the residual stenosis was 81.2% according to the WASID criteria. (**C**) Lateral view of the DSA showed that reperfusion with an mTICI of ≥2b was achieved and it was maintained for more than 20 min. (**D**). TOF-MRA performed 6 days after the operation showed a high degree of stenosis in the right MCA (black arrow). The high-resolution MRI scan on the bottom left showed an eccentric plaque (arrowhead) with enhanced stenosis that was observed at the right MCA. ICAS, intracranial atherosclerosis; NIHSS, National Institutes of Health Stroke Scale; DSA, digital subtraction angiography; MCA, middle cerebral artery; mTICI, modified thrombolysis in cerebral infarction; TOF-MRA, time of flight for magnetic resonance angiography; MRI, magnetic resonance imaging.

Table 2. Baseline characteristics and clinical outcomes of patients in Step 2 of the analysis.

	Group 1b: mTICI ≥ 2b + Stenosis < 70% (N = 61)	Group 2b: mTICI ≥ 2b + Stenosis ≥ 70% (N = 25)	p-Value
Male Sex N (%)	45 (73.8%)	17 (68.0%)	0.588
Age (mean, years)	63 ± 13	65 ± 12	0.434
Smoker N (%)	30 (50.8%)	12 (48.0%)	0.811
Hypertension, N (%)	45 (78.9%)	21 (84.0%)	0.595
DM N (%)	17 (29.3%)	7 (28.0%)	0.904
Atrial fibrillation N (%)	0 (0%)	1 (4.0%)	0.291
TIA N (%)	1 (1.6%)	1 (4.0%)	0.499
Admission NIHSS (median, IQR)	14 (11,17)	14 (10,20)	0.681
Onset-to-puncture time N (%)			0.982
Within 8 h	35 (57.4%)	15 (60.0%)	
8–24 h	26 (42.6%)	10 (40.0%)	
Good collateral flow, N (%)			0.627
ASITN ≥ 3	35 (58.3%)	16 (64.0%)	
sICH N (%)	0 (0%)	1 (4.0%)	0.298
Good prognosis N (%)	41 (67.2%)	16 (64.0%)	0.805
Mortality N (%)	0 (0%)	1 (4.0%)	0.291
Delayed reocclusion N (%)	0 (0%)	2 (8.0%)	0.082

mTICI, modified thrombolysis in cerebral infarction; DM, diabetes mellitus; TIA, transient ischemic attack; NIHSS, National Institutes of Health Stroke Scale; IQR, interquartile range; ASITN, American Society of Interventional and Therapeutic Neuroradiology collateral grading system; sICH, symptomatic intracranial hemorrhage.

3.3. Subgroup Analysis

In addition, in the group of patients who had successful thrombectomy reperfusion but severe stenosis ($n = 30$, Group 2a from Step 1), 13 patients received the rescue treatment and 12 out of the 13 patients resulted in mild to moderate residual stenosis afterwards, whereas 17 patients did not receive any rescue treatment and remained with severe residual stenosis after the EVT procedure. If we compare the 12 patients with residual stenosis management with the 17 patients without any management, the delayed reocclusion rate showed no significant difference (0/12 vs. 2/17, $p = 0.510$) and the favorable functional outcome rate showed no significant difference (6/12 vs. 12/17, $p = 0.461$).

4. Discussion

The main finding of this study is that reocclusion of the treated artery is fairly low in MCA ICAS-related occlusion patients with successful reperfusion through endovascular therapy, even with a high degree of residual stenosis after endovascular therapy. The reocclusion occurrence of ICAS patients is related to unsuccessful reperfusion rather than the severity of residual stenosis.

The findings of this study are consistent with a previous study on a Korean population [16]. In the previous study, within ICAS patients, the reocclusion rate was not found to be related to residual stenosis severity, but was influenced by reperfusion status. For patients with successful reperfusion, the reocclusion rate was much lower than that for patients without successful reperfusion (6.6% vs. 30.8%). In addition, for patients with residual stenosis, both the Korean study and this study showed a very much lower reocclusion rate after successful reperfusion. One possible explanation is the use of tirofiban. Studies [5,17] have shown that tirofiban, when delivered intra-arterially during a procedure, could dramatically reduce instant reocclusion during an endovascular procedure (85.7% reduction) as well as delayed reclusion on follow-up imaging (>70% reduction). Compared with the previous study, our study shows an even lower reocclusion rate with successful reperfusion. In this study, the tirofiban treatment was intravenously administered earlier, before the endovascular procedure, and its antiplatelet efficacy might be further improved [17]. The intravenous administration of tirofiban might also explain the low intracranial hemorrhagic rate in this study [18]. In summary, this study indicates that intravenous tirofiban treatment might be an effective treatment to prevent reocclusion and improve the success rate of endovascular treatment in ICAS patients.

The findings of our study support the use of rescue strategies, including stenting and/or angioplasty, in order to achieve successful reperfusion. However, stenting or angioplasty should be performed with caution if the aim is to address residual stenosis. It is still controversial whether stenting or angioplasty should be performed to address residual stenosis, according to the findings from previous studies [19–21]. The results of this study indicate that when successful reperfusion has been achieved, it might not be necessary to further perform stenting or angioplasty, even for patients with severe residual stenosis. It might not bring benefits but cause the following harms instead: (1) the procedure-related complication rate might increase with more endovascular operations [21,22], including the increased risk of perforating branch occlusions through emergent angioplasty; (2) the intracranial hemorrhage rate might increase with more endovascular operations [21,22], resulting from ischemic and reperfusion injuries to brain tissues [23,24], also result from intensive antiplatelet therapy after acute cerebral ischemia [25]. Furthermore, emergent angioplasty does not lower the reocclusion rate of the recanalized vessel [16,26–28] and does not improve patients' functional outcome [29]. Certainly, in light of the high reocclusion rate in the context of acute stroke with ICAS, especially in cases of high residual stenosis, we should take sufficient time to observe the blood flow changes in the target artery. In our study, the observation time was no shorter than 20 min.

The limitations of our study include the following. First, this is a retrospective single-center study with relatively small number of patients. The baseline characteristics were balanced among groups, except for the onset-to-groin puncture time. The onset-to-puncture time might be related to reocclusion rate. This confounding factor needs to be further explored in future studies. Second, the definition of ICAS might include patients with residual stenosis due to dissection or residual thrombi. Therefore, in this study, high-resolution magnetic resonance imaging was performed to confirm the diagnosis of ICAS. However, only a subgroup of patients underwent high-resolution magnetic resonance imaging. Third, the findings of this study are probably more applicable to an Asian population with a high prevalence of ICAS and are limited to middle cerebral artery occlusion.

5. Conclusions

For acute ischemic stroke resulting from intracranial artery ICAS-related occlusion, endovascular treatment should focus on increasing successful reperfusion rather than recanalization of residual stenosis.

Author Contributions: Conceptualization, T.Y., A.Z., W.C., L.L. and M.P.; data curation, Y.L., X.Z., Z.P., X.L., D.L. and R.C.; formal analysis, L.L., Y.W. and Z.P.; methodology, T.Y., A.Z., W.C. and L.L.; writing—original draft, T.Y.; writing—review and editing, W.C. and L.L. All authors have read and agreed to the published version of the manuscript.

Funding: This research was funded by the National Health commission capacity building and continuing education center, grant number GWJJ2021100203.

Institutional Review Board Statement: This study was approved by the ethics committee of Zhangzhou Affiliated Hospital of Fujian Medical University (number ID 2021 LWB227).

Informed Consent Statement: Informed consent was obtained from all subjects involved in the study.

Data Availability Statement: Not applicable.

Conflicts of Interest: The authors declare no conflict of interest.

References

1. Powers, W.J.; Rabinstein, A.A.; Ackerson, T.; Adeoye, O.M.; Bambakidis, N.C.; Becker, K.; Biller, J.; Brown, M.; Demaerschalk, B.M.; Hoh, B.; et al. 2018 Guidelines for the Early Management of Patients With Acute Ischemic Stroke: A Guideline for Healthcare Professionals From the American Heart Association/American Stroke Association. *Stroke* **2018**, *49*, e46–e110. [CrossRef] [PubMed]
2. Langhorne, P.; Ramachandra, S. Organised Inpatient (Stroke Unit) Care for Stroke: Network Meta-Analysis. *Cochrane Database Syst. Rev.* **2020**, *2020*, CD000197.
3. Mosimann, P.J.; Kaesmacher, J.; Gautschi, D.; Bellwald, S.; Panos, L.; Piechowiak, E.; Dobrocky, T.; Zibold, F.; Mordasini, P.; El-Koussy, M.; et al. Predictors of Unexpected Early Reocclusion after Successful Mechanical Thrombectomy in Acute Ischemic Stroke Patients. *Stroke* **2018**, *49*, 2643–2651. [CrossRef] [PubMed]
4. Kim, G.E.; Yoon, W.; Kim, S.K.; Kim, B.C.; Heo, T.W.; Baek, B.H.; Lee, Y.Y.; Yim, N.Y. Incidence and Clinical Significance of Acute Reocclusion after Emergent Angioplasty or Stenting for Underlying Intracranial Stenosis in Patients with Acute Stroke. *Am. J. Neuroradiol.* **2016**, *37*, 1690–1695. [CrossRef]
5. Kang, D.-H.; Kim, Y.-W.; Hwang, Y.-H.; Park, S.-P.; Kim, Y.-S.; Baik, S.K. Instant Reocclusion Following Mechanical Thrombectomy of in Situ Thromboocclusion and the Role of Low-Dose Intra-Arterial Tirofiban. *Cerebrovasc. Dis.* **2014**, *37*, 350–355. [CrossRef]
6. Heo, J.H.; Lee, K.Y.; Kim, S.H.; Kim, D.I. Immediate Reocclusion Following a Successful Thrombolysis in Acute Stroke: A Pilot Study. *Neurology* **2003**, *60*, 1684–1687. [CrossRef]
7. Jame, S.; Barnes, G. Stroke and Thromboembolism Prevention in Atrial Fibrillation. *Heart* **2020**, *106*, 10–17. [CrossRef]
8. Yi, T.Y.; Chen, W.H.; Wu, Y.M.; Zhang, M.F.; Chen, Y.H.; Wu, Z.Z.; Shi, Y.C.; Chen, B.L. Special Endovascular Treatment for Acute Large Artery Occlusion Resulting From Atherosclerotic Disease. *World Neurosurg.* **2017**, *103*, 65–72. [CrossRef]
9. Liang, W.; Wang, Y.; Du, Z.; Mang, J.; Wang, J. Intraprocedural Angiographic Signs Observed During Endovascular Thrombectomy in Patients With Acute Ischemic Stroke: A Systematic Review. *Neurology* **2021**, *96*, 1080–1090. [CrossRef]
10. Lee, J.S.; Hong, J.M.; Lee, K.S.; Suh, H.I.; Demchuk, A.M.; Hwang, Y.H.; Kim, B.M.; Kim, J.S. Endovascular Therapy of Cerebral Arterial Occlusions: Intracranial Atherosclerosis versus Embolism. *J. Stroke Cerebrovasc. Dis.* **2015**, *24*, 2074–2080. [CrossRef]
11. Yi, T.Y.; Chen, W.H.; Wu, Y.M.; Zhang, M.F.; Zhan, A.L.; Chen, Y.H.; Wu, Z.Z.; Shi, Y.C.; Chen, B.L. Microcatheter "First-Pass Effect" Predicts Acute Intracranial Artery Atherosclerotic Disease-Related Occlusion. *Neurosurgery* **2018**, *84*, 1296–1305. [CrossRef] [PubMed]
12. Chen, W.H.; Yi, T.Y.; Zhan, A.L.; Wu, Y.M.; Lu, Y.Y.; Li, Y.M.; Pan, Z.N.; Lin, D.L.; Lin, X.H. Stent-Unsheathed Effect Predicts Acute Distal Middle Cerebral Artery Atherosclerotic Disease-Related Occlusion. *J. Neurol. Sci.* **2020**, *416*, 116957. [CrossRef] [PubMed]

13. Zaidat, O.O.; Yoo, A.J.; Khatri, P.; Tomsick, T.A.; Von Kummer, R.; Saver, J.L.; Marks, M.P.; Prabhakaran, S.; Kallmes, D.F.; Fitzsimmons, B.F.M.; et al. Recommendations on Angiographic Revascularization Grading Standards for Acute Ischemic Stroke: A Consensus Statement. *Stroke* **2013**, *44*, 2650–2663. [CrossRef]
14. López-Cancio, E.; Matheus, M.G.; Romano, J.G.; Liebeskind, D.S.; Prabhakaran, S.; Turan, T.N.; Cotsonis, G.A.; Lynn, M.J.; Rumboldt, Z.; Chimowitz, M.I.; et al. Infarct Patterns, Collaterals and Likely Causative Mechanisms of Stroke in Symptomatic Intracranial Atherosclerosis. *Cerebrovasc. Dis.* **2014**, *37*, 417–422. [CrossRef] [PubMed]
15. Rocco, A.; Sallustio, F.; Toschi, N.; Rizzato, B.; Legramante, J.; Ippoliti, A.; Marchetti, A.A.; Pampana, E.; Gandini, R.; Diomedi, M. Carotid Artery Stent Placement and Carotid Endarterectomy: A Challenge for Urgent Treatment after Stroke—Early and 12-Month Outcomes in a Comprehensive Stroke Center. *J. Vasc. Interv. Radiol.* **2018**, *29*, 1254–1261. [CrossRef]
16. Hwang, Y.H.; Kim, Y.W.; Kang, D.H.; Kim, Y.S.; Liebeskind, D.S. Impact of Target Arterial Residual Stenosis on Outcome after Endovascular Revascularization. *Stroke* **2016**, *47*, 1850–1857. [CrossRef]
17. Yan, Z.; Shi, Z.; Wang, Y.; Zhang, C.; Cao, J.; Ding, C.; Qu, M.; Xia, Y.; Cai, J.; Zhang, X.; et al. Efficacy and Safety of Low-Dose Tirofiban for Acute Intracranial Atherosclerotic Stenosis Related Occlusion with Residual Stenosis after Endovascular Treatment. *J. Stroke Cerebrovasc. Dis.* **2020**, *29*, 104619. [CrossRef]
18. Yang, J.; Wu, Y.; Gao, X.; Bivard, A.; Levi, C.R.; Parsons, M.W.; Lin, L. Intraarterial Versus Intravenous Tirofiban as an Adjunct to Endovascular Thrombectomy for Acute Ischemic Stroke. *Stroke* **2020**, *51*, 2925–2933. [CrossRef]
19. Al Hasan, M.; Murugan, R. Stenting versus Aggressive Medical Therapy for Intracranial Arterial Stenosis: More Harm than Good. *Crit. Care.* **2012**, *16*, 310. [CrossRef]
20. Wakhloo, A.; Gupta, R.; Kirshner, H.; Megerian, J.T.; Lesko, J.; Pitzer, P. Effect of a Balloon-Expandable Intracranial Stent vs Medical Therapy on Risk of Stroke in Patients With Symptomatic Intracranial Stenosis. *VISSIT Randomized Clin. Trial* **2015**, *53226*, 1240–1248.
21. Alexander, M.J.; Zauner, A.; Chaloupka, J.C.; Baxter, B.; Callison, R.C.; Gupta, R.; Song, S.S.; Yu, W.; WEAVE Trial Investigators. WEAVE Trial: Final results in 152 on-label patients. *Stroke* **2019**, *50*, 889–894. [CrossRef] [PubMed]
22. Dumont, T.M.; Kan, P.; Snyder, K.V.; Hopkins, L.N.; Siddiqui, A.H.; Levy, E.I. Revisiting Angioplasty without Stenting for Symptomatic Intracranial Atherosclerotic Stenosis after the Stenting and Aggressive Medical Management for Preventing Recurrent Stroke in Intracranial Stenosis (SAMMPRIS) Study. *Neurosurgery* **2012**, *71*, 1103–1110. [CrossRef] [PubMed]
23. Piccardi, B.; Arba, F.; Nesi, M.; Palumbo, V.; Nencini, P.; Giusti, B.; Sereni, A.; Gadda, D.; Moretti, M.; Fainardi, E.; et al. Reperfusion Injury after Ischemic Stroke Study (RISKS): Single-Centre (Florence, Italy), Prospective Observational Protocol Study. *BMJ Open* **2018**, *5*, e021183.
24. Khatri, R.; McKinney, A.M.; Swenson, B.; Janardhan, V. Blood-Brain Barrier, Reperfusion Injury, and Hemorrhagic Transformation in Acute Ischemic Stroke. *Neurology* **2012**, *79*, S52–S57. [CrossRef] [PubMed]
25. Bath, P.M.; Woodhouse, L.J.; Appleton, J.P.; Beridze, M.; Christensen, H.; Dineen, R.A.; Duley, L.; England, T.J.; Flaherty, K.; Havard, D.; et al. Antiplatelet Therapy with Aspirin, Clopidogrel, and Dipyridamole versus Clopidogrel Alone or Aspirin and Dipyridamole in Patients with Acute Cerebral Ischaemia (TARDIS): A Randomised, Open-Label, Phase 3 Superiority Trial. *Lancet* **2018**, *391*, 850–859. [CrossRef]
26. Lescher, S.; Czeppan, K.; Porto, L.; Singer, O.C.; Berkefeld, J. Acute Stroke and Obstruction of the Extracranial Carotid Artery Combined with Intracranial Tandem Occlusion: Results of Interventional Revascularization. *Cardiovasc. Intervent. Radiol.* **2015**, *38*, 304–313. [CrossRef] [PubMed]
27. CChang, Y.; Kim, B.M.; Bang, O.Y.; Baek, J.H.; Heo, J.H.; Nam, H.S.; Kim, Y.D.; Yoo, J.; Kim, D.J.; Jeon, P.; et al. Rescue Stenting for Failed Mechanical Thrombectomy in Acute Ischemic Stroke a Multicenter Experience. *Stroke* **2018**, *49*, 958–964. [CrossRef]
28. Wu, C.; Chang, W.; Wu, D.; Wen, C.; Zhang, J.; Xu, R.; Liu, X.; Lian, Y.; Xie, N.; Li, C.; et al. Angioplasty and/or Stenting after Thrombectomy in Patients with Underlying Intracranial Atherosclerotic Stenosis. *Neuroradiology* **2019**, *61*, 1073–1081. [CrossRef]
29. Tsang, A.C.O.; Orru, E.; Klostranec, J.M.; Yang, I.H.; Lau, K.K.; Tsang, F.C.P.; Lui, W.M.; Pereira, V.M.; Krings, T. Thrombectomy Outcomes of Intracranial Atherosclerosis-Related Occlusions: A Systematic Review and Meta-Analysis. *Stroke* **2019**, *50*, 1460–1466. [CrossRef]

Article

Neurological Erdheim–Chester Disease Manifesting with Subacute or Progressive Cerebellar Ataxia: Novel Case Series and Review of the Literature

Vittorio Riso [1,2,†], Tommaso Filippo Nicoletti [1,3,†], Salvatore Rossi [1], Maria Gabriella Vita [4], Perna Alessia [1], Daniele Di Natale [1] and Gabriella Silvestri [1,4,*]

1. Department of Neuroscience, Neurology Section, Università Cattolica del Sacro Cuore, 20123 Rome, Italy
2. Dipartimento di Neuroscienze, UOC Neurologia, Ospedale Belcolle, 01100 Viterbo, Italy
3. Department of Neurology, University Hospital Zurich, 8091 Zurich, Switzerland
4. UOC Neurologia, Fondazione Policlinico Universitario A. Gemelli IRCCS, 20123 Rome, Italy
* Correspondence: gabriella.silvestri@unicatt.it
† These authors contributed equally to this work.

Abstract: Neurological involvement is relatively common in Erdheim–Chester disease (ECD), a rare clonal disorder of histiocytic myeloid precursors characterized by multisystem involvement. In ECD patients, neurological symptoms can occur either at onset or during the disease course and may lead to various degrees of neurological disability or affect patients' life expectancy. The clinical neurological presentation of ECD often consists of cerebellar symptoms, showing either a subacute or progressive course. In this latter case, patients manifest with a slowly progressive cerebellar ataxia, variably associated with other non-specific neurological signs, infratentorial leukoencephalopathy, and cerebellar atrophy, possibly mimicking either adult-onset degenerative or immune-mediated ataxia. In such cases, diagnosis of ECD may be particularly challenging, yet some peculiar features are helpful to address it. Here, we retrospectively describe four novel ECD patients, all manifesting cerebellar symptoms at onset. In two cases, slow disease progression and associated brain MRI features simulated a degenerative cerebellar ataxia. Three patients received a definite diagnosis of histiocytosis, whereas one case lacked histology confirmation, although clinical diagnostic features were strongly suggestive. Our findings regarding existing literature data focused on neurological ECD will be also discussed to highlight those diagnostic clues helpful to address diagnosis.

Keywords: Erdheim–Chester disease; histiocytosis; neurohistiocytosis; cerebellar ataxia

1. Introduction

The term histiocytosis refers to rare, clonal neoplasms derived from macrophage/dendritic cell lineages, giving rise to mutated monocytes [1]: according to the currently proposed pathogenic model, these cells are released in the bloodstream, and then reach the peripheral tissues, where they differentiate into foamy histiocytes eventually causing organ damage, either directly by colonization or indirectly by triggering a pro-inflammatory cascade [2].

Histiocytoses usually affect various tissues and organs, including the bone, the kidney and related retroperitoneal space, the lung, the skin, and the cardiocirculatory and the central nervous systems [1–3]. They can either affect children or adults, with differences in individual tissue involvement and histological subtype [4]. According to the most recent classification, five different main forms of histiocytosis are known: (1) Langerhans-related, (2) cutaneous and mucocutaneous, (3) malignant histiocytosis, (4) Rosai–Dorfman disease, and (5) hemophagocytic lymphohistiocytosis and macrophage activation syndrome [2]. Of note, the first group includes both Langerhans cell histiocytosis (LCH) and Erdheim–Chester disease (ECD), previously recognized as distinct entities; nearly 20% of ECD patients also present LCH lesions, and both forms are often associated with clonal pathogenic variants in genes of the MAPK pathway [2–7]. LCH mostly occurs in young patients, and ECD in adults; both affect similar brain areas manifesting with related symptomatology [4].

The clinical spectrum of ECD is heterogeneous, ranging from organ-limited (i.e., asymptomatic bone involvement) to disseminated, life-threatening forms; infiltrative lesions commonly involve the long bones determining areas of osteosclerosis, skin (xanthelasma-like lesions), retroperitoneum (peri-renal fat infiltration), cardiovascular system (peri-aortic infiltration, right atrium pseudotumor), orbits (exophthalmos), lungs, hypothalamic–pituitary involvement (diabetes insipidus), and the brain [8–12].

In most retrospective studies, clinical signs or symptoms of CNS involvement have been reported in about 40% of ECD patients [13], and in about 25% of the cases they represent the onset and/or the only clinical manifestation of ECD. Overall, brain MRI lesions are detected in more than two-thirds of patients [11], and their prevalence increases to 92% when considering ECD patients with neurological symptoms [13,14]. The clinical presentation of neurological ECD depends both on the site and the type of lesion, but progressive cerebellar and pyramidal symptoms are the most frequent, as CNS lesions in ECD more often affect the cerebellum and the brainstem. Three distinct brain MRI patterns have been recognized in ECD [15]: (i) an infiltrative pattern, with widespread lesions, nodules, or intracerebral masses, mainly involving both cerebellar and brainstem white matter, often without edema or contrast enhancement, (ii) a meningeal pattern with pseudo-granulomatous lesions involving the dura or meningioma-like lesions, and (iii) a composite pattern. Infiltrative lesions of the skull or the pituitary region, and variable signs of atrophy or iron deposition are also not infrequent [13–16]. Overall, addressing a diagnosis of neurological ECD may be challenging, particularly in patients with isolated CNS involvement manifesting with degenerative-like ataxia phenotypes: therefore, in order to dissect this topic, we describe the results of a retrospective study on a series of four novel neurological ECD patients diagnosed at our Neurological Center between 2009 and 2018. All of them presented with either subacute or chronic cerebellar symptoms associated with prominent infratentorial lesions classified as of unknown etiology. Results will be also discussed in view of available literature.

2. Materials and Methods

2.1. Patients

We retrospectively reviewed clinical, radiological, and laboratory data of four adult ECD patients (Pts #1–4, age range 52–66 years) diagnosed at the Neurological Unit of Fondazione Policlinico A. Gemelli IRCCS, Rome (Italy) between January 2009 and November 2018. The study was carried out in compliance with the Declaration of Helsinki and approved by the local ethics committee; all patients gave a written informed consent authorizing the storage and use of clinical data also for research studies.

In all patients, neurological ECD manifested with symptoms of cerebellar and/or brainstem involvement and related structural brain MRI lesions of undefined nature. An extensive diagnostic assessment documented typical extra-neurological features of ECD in all patients, and diagnosis of neurological ECD was confirmed in three patients by histopathology studies, whereas based on available clinical and diagnostic findings, the fourth patient was strongly suspected to have ECD.

2.2. Radiological Assessment

All patients underwent at least one conventional brain MR imaging study with contrast medium (gadolinium) on a 1.5 Tesla. All patients also underwent whole skeletal X-rays of upper and lower limbs. Three patients also received technetium 99-metastable (99mTc) bone scintigraphy and thoraco-abdominal CT scans with and without contrast medium, and two of them also underwent whole-body (18F)-fluorodeoxyglucose (FDG) PET.

2.3. Laboratory Assessment

All patients underwent blood cell count, electrolytes, liver and kidney function tests, serum and urine osmolality, FSH, LH, testosterone/estradiol, ACTH, cortisol, TSH, fT4, prolactin, IGF-1, C-reactive protein (CRP), erythrocyte sedimentation rate (ESR), and serum electrophoresis. CSF examination included chemical, microbiological, and cytology analyses. All patients with more progressive forms also performed an extensive screening for systemic autoimmune markers (including ANA, ENA screen, anti-dsDNA, rheumatoid factor, p-ANCA, and c-ANCA), antigliadin, and anti-onconeural antibodies. Finally, molecular testing for SCA1, 2, and FXTAS was performed in the two patients with a slowly progressive course (Pts 3 and 4).

2.4. Other Neurological Diagnostic Tests

Cognitive functions were assessed by the Mini-Mental State Examination [17] and by the Mental Deterioration Battery [18]. For three out of four patients, upper and lower limb somatosensory (SSEP) and motor evoked potentials (MEP), electromyography, and nerve conduction studies were performed.

2.5. Histopathology

Three patients (Pts 1–3) underwent diagnostic tissue biopsies from femoral, cerebellar and tibial lesions respectively, under general anesthesia: formalin-fixed paraffin-embedded tissues samples were then processed for diagnostic histopathology, including immunohistochemistry for S100, SMA, CK, AE1/AE3, CD45, CD68, CD1a, CD117, CD207, CD21, CD23, MPO, GFAP, desmin, EMA, and OLIG2, and reviewed by experienced pathologists. Iliac crest bone marrow needle aspiration and biopsy were also performed in Pts 1 and 2.

3. Results

3.1. Clinical Features

Demographic, clinical, and diagnostic data of the four ECD patients are summarized in Table 1. All patients were Caucasian; 75% were male. The median age at the onset of symptoms was 60.2 years (range 52–66 years). The mean follow-up duration was 4.62 years (standard deviation 3.51 years, range 1–8 years).

All patients manifested with either subacute or slowly progressive cerebellar symptoms mainly consisting of gait ataxia and dysarthria; three patients (75%), had also upper limb dysmetria and gaze-evoked nystagmus, and instability for subjective vertigo and ophthalmoparesis were evident in one patient (25%).

Pyramidal signs were also present in one patient (25%) who showed a mild right brachiocrural hemiparesis, and two patients (50%) had brisk deep tendon reflexes, and showed presented variable signs of involvement of cranial nerves (VII, VIII, and X).

Extrapyramidal signs were evident in two patients (50%).

Cognitive impairment in the form of attention/dysexecutive deficit was evident in one patient (25%) at the onset of symptoms.

Notably, pseudobulbar affect appeared very early in the clinical course of all three patients with more progressive symptoms.

Two patients (Pts 1 and 4) were lost to long-term follow-up, although Pt 1, who was treated by conventional chemotherapy after diagnosis of ECD, was noted to be neurologically stable after two years.

Patient 2 is currently in follow-up. He is now not able to maintain either standing or sitting positions and recently manifested seizures that were controlled by levetiracetam. His last neurological examination documented severe spastic ataxia, with marked right hemiparesis, axial, and appendicular ataxia, nystagmus, and cerebellar dysarthria, partially due to neurological sequelae after a diagnosis of cerebellar histiocytic sarcoma and related treatment.

Table 1. Summary of the demographic, main clinical, and diagnostic features documented in our case series and related treatment strategies.

Pt#, Sex	AAO	AE	Neurological	Other Neurological Findings	Skeletal Involvement	Brain MRI	Hystopathology	Treatment	Follow-Up
1,M	52	52	Dysarthria, gait ataxia, subjective dizziness	Parkinsonism, right lateropulsion in Romberg test, gaze-evoked horizontal nystagmus, eyelids ptosis, pseudobulbar affect	Area of osteosclerosis in diaphyseal bones with diffuse 18-FDG uptake	*Infiltrative pattern:* T2/FLAIR hyperintensity in MCP, pons, DN and GP without CE. Iron deposits in GP, DN and SN bilaterally.	*Left tibia biopsy:* Fibrosis with numerous macrophages, some of them foamy, and lymphocytes CD68+/CD45+, S100-, CD1a-, CD117-, CD207-. Immunochemistry for BRAFV600E-.	Subcutaneous Cladribine.	2 years, stable. Then lost at the follow-up.
2,M	60	60	Dysarthria, gait ataxia	Right lateropulsion in Romberg position, gaze-evoked rotational nystagmus, bilateral dysmetria, right hemiparesis	Diffuse osteosclerosis (vertebral body D10, left fifth rib and femur heads) with diffuse 18-FDG uptake	*Composite pattern:* T2/FLAIR hyperintensity in cerebellar hemispheres, MCP, left SCP, pons, bulb, posterior arm of IC. Two nodular areas in right cerebellar hemisphere with hypointensity in long-TR scan and with CE. Small areas of CE in the pons and in the right MCP	*Cerebellar biopsy:* Numerous histiocytes often multinucleated and with cytoplasmic vacuolation. CD 68+, S100-, CD 207-, CD1a-. Fibrosis with CD45+ lymphocytes. Conclusions: histiocytic sarcoma.	Temozolomide, autologous stem cells transplantation (FEAM protocol)	4 years, stable. Last PET-TC negative.
3,M	63	64	Dysarthria, gait imbalance, cognitive impairment	Trunkal ataxia, ophthalmoparesis, gaze-evoked nystagmus, brisk deep tendon reflexes, bilateral dysmetria, upper limbs dystonia, pseudobulbar affect.	Areas of osteosclerosis in diaphyseal bones of the 4 limbs, and II rib. Frontal sinus osteoma. Bone uptake in Tc99m scintigraphy.	*Infiltrative pattern:* T2/FLAIR hyperintensity in pons and midbrain with CE. T1 hyperintensity of pallidus nuclei. Cerebellar atrophy and iron deposits in striatal nuclei. Empty sella.	*Femur biopsy:* numerous macrophages/histiocytes CD68+ and PGM1+, S100-, SMA-.	High-dose steroid pulse therapy followed by oral maintenance therapy	6 years, worsening of ataxia and cognition, dysphagia. Death for respiratory complications.
4,F	66	76	Dysarthria, dysphonia, progressive right facial nerve peripheral palsy. Gait ataxia later	Slowing of saccadic movements, brisk deep tendon reflexes, bilateral dysmetria, pseudobulbar affect.	None	*Infiltrative pattern:* T2/FLAIR hyperintensity in pons, midbrain, cerebellum, periaqueductal and parahippocampal areas without CE. Iron deposits in GP.	Not done.	None	10 years, then lost. During follow-up: dysphagia.

Abbreviations: AAO = age at onset; AE = age at the first neurological examination; MCP = middle cerebellar peduncles; SCP = superior cerebellar peduncle; DN = dentate nuclei; GP = globus pallidus; SN = substantia nigra; CE = contrast enhancement; IC = internal capsule.

Patient 3 manifested during the follow-up a mild worsening of cerebellar ataxia and cognitive functions at neuropsychological tests. He eventually died of pneumonia six years after the onset of symptoms.

Patient 4, who had the longest period of follow-up (8 years), had moderate swallowing disturbances eight years after the initial assessment postulating a diagnosis of neurological ECD.

3.2. Laboratory Examinations

Cell blood count was normal in all patients, as well as electrolytes, liver, and renal function tests, except for slight elevated creatinine level in Pt 1, who also had increased blood IgE (506 UI/mL) and low-titer positive anti-ANA antibodies (1:160 dilution). Pituitary function and other immunological tests were normal in all cases. The CSF examination revealed slightly increased protein levels only in Pts 3 and 4, while other chemical parameters, microbiological and immunological analyses were otherwise unremarkable in all patients (Table 1).

3.3. Neuroimaging

Brain MRI showed T2/FLAIR hyperintense signal alterations without contrast enhancement variably involving the white matter of cerebellar hemispheres, middle cerebellar peduncles, dentate nuclei, pons, and midbrain and cerebral peduncles in all cases (Figure 1). Three patients (Pts 1, 2, 4) also presented similar supratentorial T2/FLAIR hyperintensities variably involving the paratrigonal area, posterior arm of the internal capsule, globus pallidus, peri-aqueductal, and parahippocampal areas, with evidence of gadolinium contrast enhancement in the paratrigonal area not shown in Pt 3. Moreover, signs of cerebellar atrophy and bilateral hypointense signal abnormalities in basal ganglia on SWI sequences, suggestive of iron deposition, were evident in Pts 1, 3, and 4 (Figure 1). Of note, in Pt 2 manifesting a subacute neurological outcome, MRI also showed two nodular lesions ($30 \times 20 \times 20$ mm^3) in the right cerebellar hemisphere with contrast enhancement (Figure 2) and elevated levels of r-CBV (regional cerebral blood volume) on the perfusion study and DWI-restriction, indicative of hypercellularity. Finally, Pt 3, affected by diabetes insipidus, also presented an empty sella. Signs of paranasal sinuses or mastoid inflammation were evident in three patients (Pts 1, 2, and 3). Spinal cord MRI was normal in all patients.

3.4. Neurophysiology

SEP and MEP documented damage of both central sensory and motor pathways in all patients. Electromyography and nerve conduction studies were normal in two out of three patients assessed, whereas in the other patient (Pt 2), also affected by diabetes mellitus type 2, documented a mild predominantly demyelinating lower limb polyneuropathy.

3.5. Cognitive Studies

Regarding cognition, initial diagnostic evaluation in Pt 1 manifested impairment in attention, executive, memory, and language (verbal fluency); similarly, Pt 4 presented a mild impairment in the same cognitive domains. In Pts 3 and 4, cognitive test were initially normal, and a serial evaluation three years later documented only in Pt 3 a moderate worsening in attention, and executive, memory, and language functions (verbal fluency). Finally, Pt 2 showed a mild defect only in one test assessing verbal fluency at the initial cognitive assessment.

3.6. Systemic Involvement

In the differential diagnosis for ECD, all patients underwent whole-body skeletal X-ray, which showed multiple areas of bone osteosclerosis, mainly involving the diaphyseal sections of upper and lower limb long bones, ribs, and the thoracic vertebrae in three patients (Pts 1, 2, and 3) (Table 1).

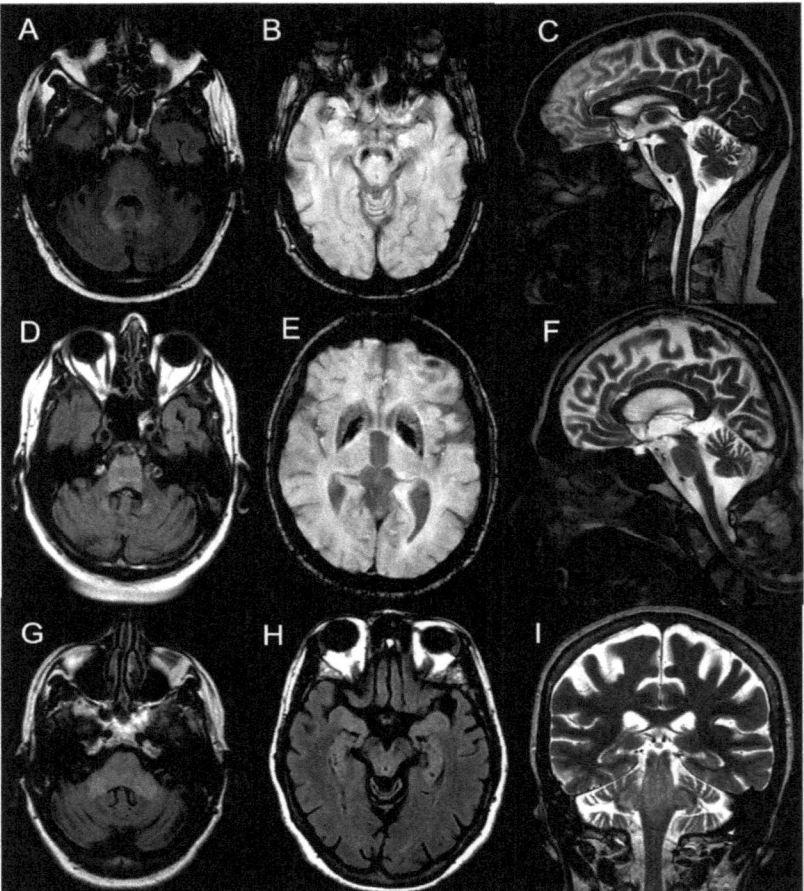

Figure 1. Panel showing brain MRI of Pt #1 (**A–C**), Pt #3 (**D–F**), and Pt #4 (**G–I**). (**A**) Transverse FLAIR scan (pons level) of Pt #1 showing mild hyperintensity of the pons, both MCPs, dentate nuclei. (**B**) Transverse SWAN scan (mesencephalon level) of Pt #1 showing marked hypointense signal (metal deposits) of bilateral substantia nigra. (**C**) Sagittal T2-weighted scan of Pt #1 showing slight vermian cerebellar atrophy. (**D**) Transverse FLAIR scan (pons level) of Pt #3 showing hyperintensity of the pons and dentate nuclei. (**E**) Transverse SWAN scan (thalami level) of Pt #3 showing marked hypointense signal (metal deposits) of putamina and globi pallidi. (**F**) Sagittal T2-weighted scan of Pt #3 showing vermian cerebellar atrophy. (**G**) Transverse FLAIR scan (pons level) of Pt #4 showing hyperintensity of the pons and both MCPs. (**H**) Transverse FLAIR scan (mesencephalon level) of Pt #4 showing hyperintensity of the mesencephalon and parahippocampal cortices. (**I**) Coronal T2-weighted scan of Pt #4 showing hyperintensity of the pons, both SCPs and MCPs. Abbreviations: Flair: fluid-attenuated inversion recovery; MCP: middle cerebellar peduncle; SWAN: susceptibility-weighted angiography; SCP: superior cerebellar peduncle.

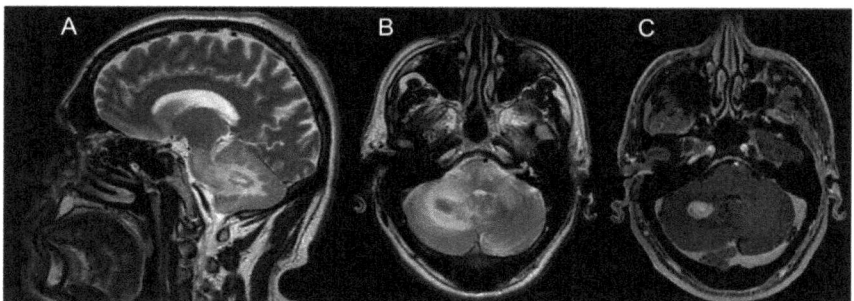

Figure 2. Panel showing brain MRI of Patient #2. (**A**) Sagittal T2-weighted scan showing one nodular lesion along with extensive hyperintensity of the white matter of the RCH, the ipsilateral MCP, and the pons. (**B**) Transverse T2-weighted scan (pons level) showing the same nodular hypointense lesion with hyperintensity of the white matter of the RCH, both MCPs and the pons. (**C**) Transverse T1-weighted scan (pons level) showing marked, homogeneous contrast enhancement of the RCH nodular lesion. Abbreviations: RCH: right cerebellar hemisphere; MCP: middle cerebellar peduncle.

These patients underwent further nuclear imaging studies (either 18-FDG CT-PET or Tc99m bone scintigraphy), all of which documented pathological uptake of the radiotracers in correspondence of the osteosclerotic lesions. Notably, increased tracer uptake was detectable in other bone sites (jaw, hip bone, vertebral column, heels) that were apparently unaffected at X-ray examination.

As previously pointed out, one patient (Pt 3) had a history of diabetes insipidus and was receiving treatment with nasal desmopressin: laboratory findings showed normal values of plasmatic and urinary osmolarity, with otherwise conserved function of the hypothalamus–hypophysis axis. Another patient (Pt 2) was affected by diabetes mellitus type 2 and treated with oral glucose-lowering agents.

A chest CT scan showed imaging features of bronchiolitis in Pt 3, while Pts 1 and 2 had a "ground glass" appearance in the lungs, also associated with slight bilateral pleural effusion and apical pleural thickening in Pt 1. Two patients (Pts 1 and 3) showed retroperitoneal fibrosis with "hairy kidney" aspect at the abdominal CT scan, although with conserved renal function. Another patient (Pt 2) had small cortical cysts bilaterally with edema of perinephric bridging septa (Table 1). An abdominal echoscan was also normal in Pt 4. Aortic parietal calcium deposits were documented in all patients.

Echocardiography was normal in all patients. Finally, eyelid xanthelasmas were evident in Pt 4.

3.7. Histopathology Data

Biopsy sites were the cerebellum in Pt 2 and the long bones in Pts 1 and 3 (tibia and femur, respectively). In all samples, numerous histiocytes were found, either multinucleated or with foamy or vacuolated cytoplasm identifiable by their immunohistochemical expression of CD68 and absence of S-100 and CD1a, which was associated with the presence of abundant fibrotic tissue or lymphoplasmacellular infiltration with positive anti-CD45 immunoreactivity. Histiocytes from Pt 1 also showed CD117 and CD207 immunoreactivity, which was instead absent in the cerebellar sample from Pt 2: in this case, mitosis and an increased proliferative index (MIB 1 = 10–15%) were also evident. According to its histopathology features, the cerebellar nodule was diagnosed as a histiocytic sarcoma.

Histochemistry for BRAFV600E was negative in the bone biopsy of Pt 1. Results of molecular testing for the BRAFV600E mutation were not available from medical records in Pt 2, while testing was negative in whole leukocytes DNA from Pt 3.

3.8. Management and Follow-Up

Following diagnosis, both Pts 1 and 2 were referred to the Division of Haematology of our Centre for Therapeutic Management and Follow-up. Pt 1 was initially treated with oral steroids without any clinical improvement and then treated with chemotherapy by subcutaneous cladribine (5 injections/month for 4–5 months). Serial PET FDG studies showed persistent reduced uptake of the radioligand in correspondence of the bone lesions during two years of follow-up.

Pt 2, diagnosed with histiocytic sarcoma, was treated with radiotherapy and chemotherapy (temozolomide 150 mg for 3 months) with poor response; thus, he underwent an autologous peripheral stem cell transplantation, preceded by a FEAM (fotemustine/aracytine/etoposide/melphalan) protocol as conditioning therapy. Serial MRI and scans showed good response to treatment, with no evidence of disease recurrence at both MRI and global PET CT scan two years after treatment.

According to their clinical histories and the results of the diagnostic work-up, both Pts 3 and 4 were diagnosed with neurodegenerative ECD. Based on the evidence of contrast enhanced lesions in the brain MRI, Pt 3 underwent a cycle of steroid pulse therapy (1 g/day for 5 days) followed by a maintenance therapy with oral corticosteroids (starting dose of prednisone 50 mg/day), which produced a temporary, partial clinical benefit on gait balance problems, with a concomitant disappearance of contrast enhancement in the brain MRI (data not shown). However, his cerebellar ataxia thereafter returned to slowly progressive despite this treatment, so steroids were tapered until suspension, without registering any significant clinical and neuroimaging worsening. Patient 4 had a very mild disease progression. In consideration of the relatively benign course, and of the potential side effects of conventional therapies, no further treatment was performed for either patient.

4. Discussion

This case series illustrates the occurrence of Erdheim–Chester disease presenting exclusively with neurological manifestations. This issue now appears important, as CNS involvement may affect the life expectancy of ECD patients [19], and recent research indicates there is a significant response of CNS symptoms to novel drugs specifically targeting the MAPK pathway [14,20], the dysregulation of which plays a main role in the pathogenesis of ECD. The relevance of CNS involvement in ECD is underlined by different systematic literature reviews, regarding both the high prevalence of neurological involvement and also of neurological presentation of ECD.

Of note, in our small ECD cohort neurological involvement remained the only clinical manifestation of ECD, consisting of subacute or progressive cerebellar and brainstem symptoms associated with prominent involvement of the infratentorial white matter on the brain MRI. A similar presentation was previously highlighted in a previous case series [21], and our findings actually support that patients with exclusive neurological ECD might represent a specific subgroup, distinct from ECD, characterized by extraneurological presentation.

According to the literature, we observed a similar male prevalence in our cohort (3M, 1F). In addition to cerebellar symptoms, the pseudobulbar effect was another common clinical feature in our ECD cohort; accordingly, in a recent review of 30 ECD patients with prominent neurological involvement, Bathia and colleagues [14] reported the presence of bulbar affect in about 30% of cases, supporting that this symptom might represent a "red flag" to suspect neurological ECD when combined with ataxia and the presence of peculiar infratentorial neuroimaging lesions.

Other neurological manifestations, such as cranial nerves involvement or diplopia, similarly occurred at a relatively low prevalence in our small ECD cohort. In addition, 50% of our patients showed clinical pyramidal signs, and in all of them, motor and sensory evoked potential documented an involvement of both long descending and ascending central pathways, likely related to the widespread white matter brainstem involvement.

A high prevalence of cognitive impairment was also documented in our cohort of neurological ECD patients, mainly affecting verbal fluency, memory, and executive functions. These findings are in agreement with those of Boyd et al. [16], who reported a similar prevalence and pattern of cognitive involvement in a cohort of 15 ECD patients assessed by a detailed neuropsychological battery. In this study, voxel-based morphometry documented significantly reduced brain volumes in ECD patients vs. healthy controls, with specific loss of grey matter in the right frontal and parietal cortex, and routine brain MRI from a larger cohort of 62 ECD patients documented signs of brain atrophy in about 20–30% of cases. These results suggest the occurrence of neurodegenerative damage in ECD brains. Accordingly, brain MRI showed both cerebellar atrophy and signs of iron deposition both in the basal ganglia and cerebellar nuclei in Pts 1, 3, and 4 with a progressive neurological disease course.

Regarding brain MRI, all our neurological ECD patients had a suggestive "infiltrative pattern", characterized by T2/FLAIR hyperintense white matter lesions mainly involving the brainstem and the cerebellum, usually without contrast enhancement. Some of them showed similar alterations also in the supratentorial compartment, in one case with focal areas of contrast enhancement. Overall, our data support those of previous reports indicating that the characteristic brain MRI findings in "pure "neurological ECD patients consists of a diffuse, exclusive, or prominent involvement of the infratentorial compartment mainly involving the cerebellum, the brainstem, and the cerebellar peduncles, usually without contrast enhancement [13–16,21] and with no evidence of meningeal involvement. As an additional diagnostic hint for ECD, diabetes insipidus had occurred in Pt 3 many years before the onset of ataxia. Such a condition is relatively frequent in ECD, being reported in 30–48% of patients, and it may occur, as in our patient, many years before the onset of neurological symptoms. A long-lasting history of diabetes insipidus associated with thickening and contrast enhancement of the pituitary stalk, in the presence of unspecific brain, meningeal, or retro-orbital lesions might also imply a differential diagnosis of IgG4-related disease, sarcoidosis, tuberculosis, or lymphocytic infundibulo-neurohypophysitis. Yet, the association with diffuse signs of long bone involvement is highly suggestive for a diagnosis of neuro-ECD, as discussed shortly after in this section. Finally, two large tumoral nodular lesions in the right cerebellar hemisphere with contrast enhancement were also present in Pt 2, who accordingly manifested rapidly evolving symptoms due to its mass effect in the posterior fossa.

Another diagnostic clue for neurological ECD might be represented by the presence of signs of sinusitis and/or mastoiditis on the brain MRI, as subclinical systemic disease manifestations, reported in about 30% of ECD patients characterized by neurohystiocitic involvement [14,21]. In this regard, however, the most suggestive extraneurological feature of ECD present in three of our patients was the presence of multiple areas of bone osteosclerosis, mainly involving the diaphyseal sections of long bones, ribs, and the thoracic vertebrae, and characterized by more widespread pathological uptake of the radiotracers at nuclear imaging studies. Asymptomatic bone lesions are reported with a very high prevalence (80–100%) in neuro-ECD cohorts [14,21,22]. However, their absence does not rule out an ECD diagnosis, as about 20–26% of ECD patients may not present signs of bone involvement [8,11].

Other typical subclinical systemic ECD signs were detected in Pts 1, 2, and 3 through thoraco-abdominal CT scans: these included signs of renal and retroperitoneal infiltration characterized by hairy kidney and ground glass appearance of lungs or pleural effusion. Moreover, eyelid xanthelasma-like lesions were detected in Pt 4. Conversely, none of our patients presented signs of periaortitis, or heart involvement.

A definite diagnosis of ECD, according to current diagnostic criteria for ECD [20] requiring histology confirmation, was reached in three patients of our cohort: in particular in Pt 2, one nodular lesion configured a histiocytic sarcoma. Histiocytic sarcoma, a malignant proliferation of cells showing signs of histiocytic differentiation, often occurring in the skin, the lymph nodes, and the intestinal tract, while primary peripheral or CNS involvement is very rare [23,24]. It has often poor prognosis, but patients with localized histiocytic sarcoma may survive years after the initial diagnosis followed by aggressive clinical management. Data from single case reports have suggested efficacy for high-dose chemotherapy and autologous/allogeneic stem cell transplantation; indeed, our patient, treated by autologous peripheral stem-cell transplantation preceded by FEAM (fotemustine/aracytine/etoposide/melphalan) protocol as conditioning therapy, shows no signs of active disease at the last CT-PET after 4 years of follow-up. In Pt 2, the presence of systemic bone manifestations, and the evidence of diffuse infratentorial brainstem and cerebellar alterations with only limited contrast enhancement at the brain MRI are both features suggestive of ECD. Thus, we suggest that both ECD and histiocytic sarcoma may coexist in this patient, originating from a common neoplastic precursor, as such disorders may share the same oncogene background [2,6,7,25,26].

In both Pts 1 and 3, bone histology confirmed ECD diagnosis. Following hematological evaluation, Pt 1 was treated by conventional chemotherapy, and we could observe a substantial neurological stability after two years of follow up; then, the patient was lost. After steroids, in agreement with hematologists, Pt 3 was not treated with further drugs, in consideration of his isolated and slowly progressive neurological involvement and the potential serious side effects of other immunosuppressive or chemotherapy drugs. Unfortunately, we did not reach a definite histological confirmation of ECD in Pt 4, yet we believe that her clinical and brain MRI features, together with the presence of skin manifestations, would strongly support an ECD diagnosis also in this case.

ECD has been associated with mutations in genes involved either in the MAPK and the P13K-AKT signaling pathways, which eventually activate cell proliferation, survival, and angiogenesis; in particular, more than 50% of the ECD patients carry somatic BRAF (V600E) gene mutation in affected tissues, that sometimes can be detected also on DNA from peripheral blood. In our retrospective data analysis, histochemical staining for BRAFV600E was reported to be negative in bone tissue biopsy of Pt 1, and molecular testing, performed only in blood DNA, was also negative in Pt 3. No molecular data regarding Pt 1 and Pt 4 were available from medical records.

Currently, molecular characterization of ECD lesions may allow the establishment of more effective chemotherapies specifically targeting the dysfunctional pathway, i.e., BRAF inhibitors vemurafenib or dabrafenib for BRAF-mutated ECD patients, and recent studies indicate that these drugs would be also successful on CNS involvement.

However, the pathogenesis of neurological damage in ECD still needs clarification: indeed, signs of cortical brain atrophy have also been documented in ECD patients without corresponding supratentorial lesions [16,27]. Further studies are needed to better clarify the pathogenesis of neurodegeneration in ECD patients, which might be either triggered by systemic inflammation secondary to histiocytic infiltration in other tissues, or by other still unknown mechanisms [2].

Author Contributions: Conceptualization, V.R., M.G.V. and G.S.; data curation, V.R., T.F.N., S.R., M.G.V., P.A., D.D.N. and G.S.; writing—original draft preparation, V.R. and T.F.N.; writing—review and editing, S.R. and G.S.; visualization, S.R.; supervision, G.S. All authors have read and agreed to the published version of the manuscript.

Funding: This research received no external funding.

Institutional Review Board Statement: The study was conducted in accordance with the Declaration of Helsinki, and approved by the Ethics Committee of Fondazione Policlinico Agostino Gemelli IRCCS.

Informed Consent Statement: Informed consent was obtained from all subjects involved in the study.

Data Availability Statement: Anonymized patients' data are available on reasonable request.

Conflicts of Interest: The authors declare no conflict of interest.

References

1. Emile, J.F.; Abla, O.; Fraitag, S.; Horne, A.; Haroche, J.; Donadieu, J.; Requena-Caballero, L.; Jordan, M.B.; Abdel-Wahab, O.; Allen, C.E.; et al. Histiocyte Society. Revised classification of histiocytoses and neoplasms of the macrophage-dendritic cell lineages. *Blood* **2016**, *127*, 2672–2681. [CrossRef] [PubMed]
2. Pegoraro, F.; Papo, M.; Maniscalco, V.; Charlotte, F.; Haroche, J.; Vaglio, A. Erdheim-Chester disease: A rapidly evolving disease model. *Leukemia* **2020**, *34*, 2840–2857. [CrossRef] [PubMed]
3. Haroche, J.; Cohen-Aubart, F.; Rollins, B.J.; Donadieu, J.; Charlotte, F.; Idbaih, A.; Vaglio, A.; Abdel-Wahab, O.; Emile, J.-F.; Amoura, Z. Histiocytoses: Emerging neoplasia behind inflammation. *Lancet Oncol.* **2017**, *18*, e113–e125. [CrossRef]
4. Diamond, E.L.; Durham, B.H.; Haroche, J.; Yao, Z.; Ma, J.; Parikh, S.A.; Wang, Z.; Choi, J.; Kim, E.; Cohen-Aubart, F.; et al. Diverse and targetable kinase alterations drive histiocytic neoplasms. *Cancer Discov.* **2016**, *6*, 154–165. [CrossRef] [PubMed]
5. Cohen Aubart, F.; Idbaih, A.; Emile, J.F.; Amoura, Z.; Abdel-Wahab, O.; Durham, B.H.; Haroche, J.; Diamond, E.L. Histiocytosis and the nervous system: From diagnosis to targeted therapies. *Neuro Oncol.* **2021**, *23*, 1433–1446. [CrossRef]
6. Haroche, J.; Charlotte, F.; Arnaud, L.; von Deimling, A.; Hélias-Rodzewicz, Z.; Hervier, B.; Cohen-Aubart, F.; Launay, D.; Lesot, A.; Mokhtari, K.; et al. High prevalence of BRAF V600E mutations in Erdheim-Chester disease but not in other non-Langerhans cell histiocytoses. *Blood* **2012**, *120*, 2700–2703. [CrossRef]
7. Emile, J.-F.; Diamond, E.L.; Hélias-Rodzewicz, Z.; Cohen-Aubart, F.; Charlotte, F.; Hyman, D.M.; Kim, E.; Rampal, R.; Patel, M.; Ganzel, C.; et al. Recurrent RAS and PIK3CA mutations in Erdheim-Chester disease. *Blood* **2014**, *124*, 3016–3019. [CrossRef]
8. Cives, M.; Simone, V.; Rizzo, F.M.; Dicuonzo, F.; Lacalamita, M.C.; Ingravallo, G.; Silvestris, F.; Dammacco, F. Erdheim-Chester disease: A systematic review. *Crit. Rev. Oncol. Hematol.* **2015**, *95*, 1–11. [CrossRef]
9. Cavalli, G.; Guglielmi, B.; Berti, A.; Campochiaro, C.; Sabbadini, M.G.; Dagna, L. The multifaceted clinical presentations and manifestations of Erdheim-Chester disease: Comprehensive review of the literature and of 10 new cases. *Ann. Rheum. Dis.* **2013**, *72*, 1691–1695. [CrossRef]
10. Mazor, R.D.; Manevich-Mazor, M.; Shoenfeld, Y. Erdheim-Chester Disease: A comprehensive review of the literature. *Orphanet. J. Rare Dis.* **2013**, *8*, 137. [CrossRef]
11. Estrada-Veras, J.I.; O'Brien, K.J.; Boyd, L.C.; Dave, R.H.; Durham, B.H.; Xi, L.; Malayeri, A.A.; Chen, M.Y.; Gardner, P.J.; Enriquez, J.R.A.; et al. The clinical spectrum of Erdheim-Chester disease: An observational cohort study. *Blood Adv.* **2017**, *1*, 357–366. [CrossRef] [PubMed]
12. Starkebaum, G.; Hendrie, P. Erdheim-Chester disease. *Best Pract. Res. Clin. Rheumatol.* **2020**, *34*, 101510. [CrossRef] [PubMed]
13. Cohen Aubart, F.; Idbaih, A.; Galanaud, D.; Law-Ye, B.; Emile, J.-F.; Charlotte, F.; Donadieu, J.; Maksud, P.; Seilhean, D.; Amoura, Z.; et al. Central nervous system involvement in Erdheim-Chester disease: An observational cohort study. *Neurology* **2020**, *95*, e2746–e2754. [CrossRef] [PubMed]
14. Bhatia, A.; Hatzoglou, V.; Ulaner, G.; Rampal, R.; Hyman, D.M.; Abdel-Wahab, O.; Durham, B.H.; Dogan, A.; Ozkaya, N.; Yabe, M.; et al. Neurologic and oncologic features of Erdheim-Chester disease: A 30-patient series. *Neuro Oncol.* **2020**, *22*, 979–992. [CrossRef] [PubMed]
15. Lachenal, F.; Cotton, F.; Desmurs-Clavel, H.; Haroche, J.; Taillia, H.; Magy, N.; Hamidou, M.; Salvatierra, J.; Piette, J.-C.; Vital-Durand, D.; et al. Neurological manifestations and neuroradiological presentation of Erdheim-Chester disease: Report of 6 cases and systematic review of the literature. *J. Neurol.* **2006**, *253*, 1267–1277. [CrossRef] [PubMed]
16. Boyd, L.C.; O'Brienm, K.J.; Ozkaya, N.; Lehky, T.; Meoded, A.; Gochuico, B.R.; Hannah-Shmouni, F.; Nath, A.; Toro, C.; Gahl, W.A.; et al. Neurological manifestations of Erdheim-Chester Disease. *Ann. Clin. Transl. Neurol.* **2020**, *7*, 497–506. [CrossRef]
17. Folstein, M.F.; Folstein, S.E.; McHugh, P.R. "Mini-mental state": A practical method for grading the cognitive state of patients for the clinician. *J. Psychiatr. Res.* **1975**, *12*, 189–198. [CrossRef]
18. Carlesimo, G.A.; Caltagirone, C.; Gainotti, G. The Mental Deterioration Battery: Normative data, diagnostic reliability and qualitative analyses of cognitive impairment. The Group for the Standardization of the Mental Deterioration Battery. *Eur. Neurol.* **1996**, *36*, 378–384. [CrossRef]
19. Arnaud, L.; Hervier, B.; Néel, A.; Hamidou, M.A.; Kahn, J.E.; Wechsler, B.B.; Pérez-Pastor, G.G.; Blomberg, B.; Fuzibet, J.-G.J.-G.; Dubourguet, F.F.; et al. CNS involvement and treatment with interferon-α are independent prognostic factors in Erdheim-Chester disease: A multicenter survival analysis of 53 patients. *Blood* **2011**, *117*, 2778–2782. [CrossRef]
20. Goyal, G.; Heaney, M.L.; Collin, M.; Cohen-Aubart, F.; Vaglio, A.; Durham, B.H.; Hershkovitz-Rokah, O.; Girschikofsky, M.; Jacobsen, E.D.; Toyama, K.; et al. Erdheim-Chester disease: Consensus recommendations for evaluation, diagnosis, and treatment in the molecular era. *Blood* **2020**, *135*, 1929–1945. [CrossRef]
21. Chiapparini, L.; Cavalli, G.; Langella, T.; Venerando, A.; De Luca, G.; Raspante, S.; Marotta, G.; Pollo, B.; Lauria, G.; Cangi, M.G.; et al. Adult leukoencephalopathies with prominent infratentorial involvement can be caused by Erdheim-Chester disease. *J. Neurol.* **2018**, *265*, 273–284. [CrossRef] [PubMed]
22. Haque, A.; Pérez, C.A.; Reddy, T.A.; Gupta, R.K. Erdheim-Chester Disease with Isolated CNS Involvement: A Systematic Review of the Literature. *Neurol. Int.* **2022**, *14*, 716–726. [CrossRef] [PubMed]
23. Schlick, K.; Aigelsreiter, A.; Pichler, M.; Reitter, S.; Neumeister, P.; Hoefler, G.; Beham-Schmid, C.; Linkesch, W. Onkologie Histiocytic sarcoma—Targeted therapy: Novel therapeutic options? A series of 4 cases. *Onkologie* **2012**, *35*, 447–450. [CrossRef] [PubMed]

24. Moulignier, A.; Mikol, J.; Heran, F.; Galicier, L. Isolated III cranial nerve palsies may point to primary histiocytic sarcoma. *BMJ Case Rep.* **2014**, *2014*, bcr2014204663. [CrossRef]
25. Shanmugam, V.; Griffin, G.K.; Jacobsen, E.D.; Fletcher, C.D.M.; Sholl, L.M.; Hornick, J.L. Identification of diverse activating mutations of the RAS-MAPK pathway in histiocytic sarcoma. *Mod. Pathol.* **2019**, *32*, 830–843. [CrossRef] [PubMed]
26. Branco, B.; Comont, T.; Ysebaert, L.; Picard, M.; Laurent, C.; Oberic, L. Targeted therapy of BRAF V600E-mutant histiocytic sarcoma: A case report and review of the literature. *Eur. J. Haematol.* **2019**, *103*, 444–448. [CrossRef]
27. Diamond, E.L.; Hatzoglou, V.; Patel, S.; Abdel-Wahab, O.; Rampal, R.; Hyman, D.M.; Holodny, A.I.; Raj, A. Diffuse reduction of cerebral grey matter volumes in Erdheim-Chester disease. *Orphanet. J. Rare Dis.* **2016**, *11*, 109. [CrossRef]

Disclaimer/Publisher's Note: The statements, opinions and data contained in all publications are solely those of the individual author(s) and contributor(s) and not of MDPI and/or the editor(s). MDPI and/or the editor(s) disclaim responsibility for any injury to people or property resulting from any ideas, methods, instructions or products referred to in the content.

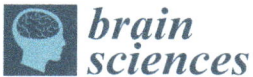

Communication

Perspective: Present and Future of Virtual Reality for Neurological Disorders

Hyuk-June Moon [1] and Sungmin Han [1,2,*]

[1] Bionics Research Center, Biomedical Research Division, Korea Institute of Science and Technology (KIST), Seoul 02792, Republic of Korea
[2] Division of Bio-Medical Science & Technology, Korea Institute of Science and Technology School, Korea University of Science and Technology (UST), Seoul 02792, Republic of Korea
* Correspondence: han0318@kist.re.kr

Abstract: Since the emergence of Virtual Reality technology, it has been adopted in the field of neurology. While Virtual Reality has contributed to various rehabilitation approaches, its potential advantages, especially in diagnosis, have not yet been fully utilized. Moreover, new tides of the Metaverse are approaching rapidly, which will again boost public and research interest and the importance of immersive Virtual Reality technology. Nevertheless, accessibility to such technology for people with neurological disorders has been critically underexplored. Through this perspective paper, we will briefly look over the current state of the technology in neurological studies and then propose future research directions, which hopefully facilitate beneficial Virtual Reality studies on a wider range of topics in neurology.

Keywords: virtual reality; neurological; cognitive; rehabilitation; diagnosis; metaverse

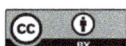

1. Introduction: Present of Virtual Reality

In the mid-2010s, with the launches of several commercial products, Virtual Reality (VR) technology attracted significant public and research attention (although, surprisingly, the origin of the technology dates back to the 1980s) [1,2]. Thanks to its immersive system, including head-mounted displays (HMDs), it has an outstanding capability to simulate lifelike experiences from the first-person perspective (1 PP). Thus, VR has been introduced to the field of psychiatric disorders, for instance, as therapy for phobias, anxiety disorders, and post-traumatic stress [3–5]. Likewise, VR has been utilized in the rehabilitation of patients with neurological disorders, motivating them to be more actively engaged and immersed via fun and game-like methods (for a review [6,7]). While VR technology has been shown to facilitate recovery and enhance motor or cognitive functions in patients with Alzheimer's disease (AD), Parkinson's disease (PD), or stroke, it has rarely been used for the diagnosis of such diseases or the evaluation of the related cognitive impairments, where it has many advantages over conventional methods. In contrast to the exaggerated expectations of the time when it first appeared, the era of VR (replacing other traditional displays) has not immediately arrived due to many obstacles: lack of affordable consumer products and enjoyable content, difficulties in dedicated software development, limited hardware performance (e.g., insufficient computing power and display resolutions, usage with bulky cables, or limited battery time), limited sensory modalities, and cybersickness (nausea, vomiting, dizziness, or fatigue) [8,9]. Along with public trends, it has also become less actively adopted in research than before, including the field of neurology. However, those obstacles are decreasing thanks to the continuous development of better and more affordable VR systems, and, at last, the recent rise of the Metaverse is about to bring the second golden age of VR technology (Figure 1).

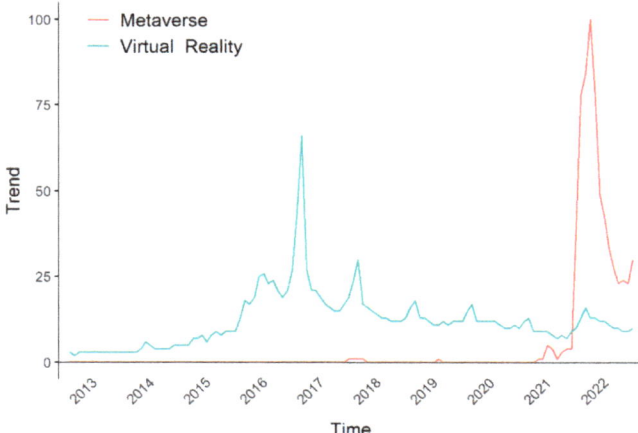

Figure 1. The results of Google Trends for 'Metaverse' and 'Virtual Reality' over time (2013 to 2022). The trends show the Virtual Reality boom in the mid-2010s and the recent emergence of the Metaverse.

At this very critical moment, through this short communication, we would like to propose ways to better utilize advanced VR technology for patients with neurological disorders (focusing on diagnosis and evaluation) and would also like to suggest future research avenues necessary for such patients to fully enjoy the era of the Metaverse together. Hopefully, this can facilitate various VR studies to benefit neurological patients. Of note, in this manuscript, VR refers to immersive VR with a stereo HMD [2], rather than the too broad definition of 'a computer-generated world'.

2. Possibility for Diagnosis or Assessment of Cognitive Impairments

Many neurological diseases accompany a wide range of cognitive impairments, which can lead to mild cognitive impairment (MCI) and even to dementia at later stages [10,11]. AD is the most common cause of dementia, and there are also other neurological diseases that can significantly impair cognitive functions, such as stroke, PD, and dementia with Lewy bodies. Various kinds of tests (for instance, the Mini-Mental State Examination (MMSE), the Montreal Cognitive Assessment (MoCA), and Mini-Cog) are currently used to assess cognitive impairments and screen such diseases [12,13]. However, those tests are often not straightforward to interpret: their results are affected by education level, language, and race/ethnicity [12,14]. Moreover, there can be ceiling or floor effects for scoring an individual category of cognitive functions, and the summed binary or ordinal score data are often analyzed as metric data, which might lead to statistically incorrect results [15]. Due to such issues, it is difficult for such tests to be used generally to diagnose various diseases and to distinguish different stages of their progression (e.g., MCI from dementia).

Hopefully, VR-based tests can serve as better assessment tools for cognitive impairments (Figure 2). First, VR can simulate situations that may occur in our daily lives (e.g., buying a list of products at the market or navigating to specific places in town) and assess the relevant cognitive abilities (e.g., working memory, executive function, spatial navigation, spatial memory, and cognitive planning) as a VR-based cognitive test. The results of such tasks can directly indicate whether subjects can adequately perform the specific tasks in their lives (so that they can request support if needed). Notably, the likely situations are shown in the 1PP through VR systems (including HMDs and sound systems), which dramatically boosts immersion in the virtual scenario (i.e., the cognitive test) and, arguably, makes the test results even more reliable.

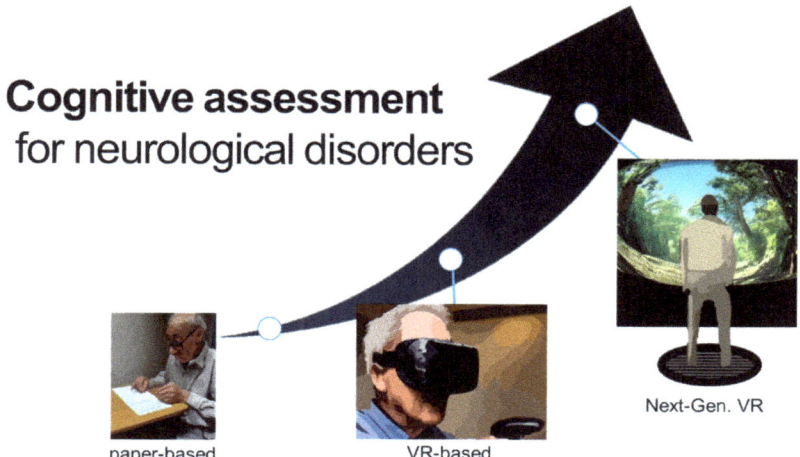

Figure 2. Cognitive assessment tools for neurological disorders will hopefully evolve from paper-based tests into next-generation VR-based tests with advances in VR technology.

In addition, not only the mere binary results of the task (i.e., success or failure) but also many detailed parameters, which might contain much richer information regarding one's cognitive functions, can be acquired during VR-based tasks. For instance, Kunz and colleagues [16] reported navigation pattern changes (i.e., a tendency to navigate closer to arena boundaries) during a spatial navigation memory task in a group with a genetic risk of AD, while their spatial memory precision did not differ from the healthy control group (arguably due to the compensatory mechanisms of intact brain regions). Likewise, many other parameters of VR tasks (e.g., navigation distance or trial time [17]) may convey information about disease-related cognitive impairments that could be missing from conventional tests.

Importantly, VR-based tests can provide unbiased and more objective test results than conventional methods (especially those using traditional displays). In VR paradigms, a virtual experimenter instead of a human instructor can give instructions, reducing any influence or bias possibly introduced by different experimenters and improving double-blind or multi-center experimental designs [18]. In addition, VR can fully control visual inputs, on which human beings largely depend [19]. HMDs can mask other visual inputs to minimize possible distractions during tests. Moreover, the size of any text or object shown to participants can be precisely controlled by stereoscopic HMDs (whereas for traditional displays, diverse screen sizes and the distance from the screen can critically affect those parameters). The control of visual input will be even more critical if cognitive tests are combined with neuroimaging since differences in visual information can significantly affect one's brain activity [20]. This can help standardize multi-center research or even allow home-based tracking of patients' cognitive abilities, which will likely promote the neurorehabilitation of life-relevant functions through repetitions of such VR tasks [6,7]. Additionally, VR with HMDs can be used to detect decreased stereopsis in PD patients [21], providing more standardized and controlled assessment methods.

3. Next-Generation VR Systems

More advanced VR systems combined with technologies from other fields (for instance, robotics, neuroscience, or materials) are promising candidates for next-generation VR paradigms that can benefit patients with neurological disorders. A recently published study by Alberts and colleagues integrated a VR system with an omnidirectional treadmill and implemented a VR grocery shopping task [22], which allowed them to assess patients' cognitive-motor functions (beyond just cognitive ones) with various detailed behavioral parameters during the task (e.g., the occurrence of freezing of gait). This study showed significant progress toward ideal VR-based testing. Such a paradigm can further assess the dual-task (or multiple-task) abilities of patients [23]. It has been shown that performing physical and cognitive tasks simultaneously (as is usually required in our daily lives) can significantly worsen individual task performance, especially when each demands a high level of attention. As expected, decreased postural control or gait performance has been reported in the elderly when presented with dual-task situations (who need to pay more attention than the young population when performing such physical tasks, as do patients with neurological disorders) [24]. Hence, such VR-motor paradigms can more accurately evaluate a patient's real-life abilities. However, despite the advantages of the VR-motor platform, the cost of the omnidirectional treadmill used in the study (Infinadeck, starting at USD 40 K according to the manufacturer's website) is not easily affordable for many clinics or research institutes (and even by individuals who can benefit from home-based VR approaches). There are also alternative omnidirectional VR treadmills with more affordable prices (USD 1~2 K), such as KAT VR or Omni One. Thus, more studies should follow to investigate whether those devices (which seem to target young people playing VR games) can also be applied to elderly individuals, especially those with various neurological conditions, in terms of usability and safety.

To develop and establish a next-generation VR-based cognitive assessment, it is first necessary to design an appropriate VR-based task based on the real-life necessary abilities or cognitive (or cognitive-motor) functions to be tested. Importantly, as mentioned above, the task parameters should be standardized as much as possible through VR systems so that the data from various studies can be integrated without problems. Then, using a VR-based task, enough data should be collected from diverse populations with different ethnicities, races, sexes/genders, and diseases (necessarily through international collaborations). The collected data should be analyzed to establish appropriate methods to quantify each category of cognitive functions. Along the way, the quantified VR task results should also be compared with other tests currently used in clinics (e.g., the MMSE and the MoCA) to validate their utility and whether they can replace conventional tests at some point (after a broad consensus is formed).

Notably, there are novel VR-based neuroscience approaches that experimentally induce hallucinations similar to psychiatric symptoms, such as out-of-body experiences [25–27]. Importantly, a recent study by Bernasconi and colleagues demonstrated that a robot-based experimental induction of a psychiatric symptom could tell whether a PD patient was experiencing such a symptom in one's daily life; presence hallucinations (from which up to 60% of PD patients suffer [28]) were more easily induced in the lab for patients with the same symptoms [29]. Such approaches combining VR and cognitive neuroscience can be further applied to diagnose neurological diseases with psychiatric symptoms (e.g., hallucinations and delusions) and to predict related prognoses.

4. The Metaverse for Patients with Neurological Disorders

We are now seeing the rise of the Metaverse (Figure 1). The term 'Metaverse' was first introduced in the science fiction novel *Snow Crash* (1992) as an immersive virtual world that users can access via a VR system [30]. Importantly, in the Metaverse, people can live as an avatar (computer-generated body, which does not necessarily resemble one's physical body) and interact with others (i.e., avatars of other people) [31]. Thanks to the advent of the internet and advanced VR systems, the Metaverse, which was only imagined three decades ago, is now about to be realized. Public and research interest in it is rapidly increasing. The Metaverse is often linked to immersive experience in virtual worlds. Accordingly, interest in VR systems that could provide a more realistic and diverse sensory experience than conventional devices is also growing again. Of note, the Metaverse can be especially beneficial for patients with neurological disorders, allowing them to freely move around and communicate with others in the virtual world, unlike in the real world. This can benefit not only patients' social/mental health (as most of us experienced during the COVID-19 pandemic [32]) but also their cognitive functions [33]. However, the digital divide, which exists now for the use of digital devices or online/internet services [34,35] and will probably become more critical for VR devices and the Metaverse, needs to be addressed so that the elderly and especially patients with neurological diseases do not fall behind. Such patients likely have brain mechanisms or functions that differ from those of the healthy population. Hence, it should be investigated whether they can access immersive VR and the Metaverse without suffering from severe cybersickness or fatigue. Furthermore, studies on how to prevent or ameliorate such VR-induced side effects, such as whether continued exposure to an immersive VR experience may alleviate or exacerbate them or whether physiological stimulation (e.g., on the vestibular system or brain) can help, should also be followed.

5. Conclusions

When VR was first introduced in the field of neurology, it was expected to open a new stage of clinical research. However, the advantages of VR have yet to be fully utilized. While the rapidly approaching tides of the Metaverse can benefit patients with neurological disorders, they will, at the same time, require them to be prepared and adapted to life in the new era, which can be even more challenging for these patients than for a healthy population. Hopefully, this paper will facilitate many future VR studies that benefit patients, providing better tools for assessing their cognitive impairments and enabling them to enjoy freer and happier lives in the Metaverse.

Author Contributions: Conceptualization, H.-J.M. and S.H.; methodology, H.-J.M.; validation, H.-J.M. and S.H.; writing—original draft preparation, H.-J.M. and S.H.; writing—review and editing, H.-J.M. and S.H.; visualization, H.-J.M.; supervision, H.-J.M. and S.H.; project administration, H.-J.M. and S.H.; funding acquisition, H.-J.M. and S.H. All authors have read and agreed to the published version of the manuscript.

Funding: This work was supported in part by the Korea Institute of Science and Technology (KIST) Institutional Program (2E31642), a National Research Council of Science & Technology (NST) grant from the South Korean government (MSIT) (CAP-18015-000), and the Smart HealthCare program (www.kipot. or. Kr, 5 December 2022) (220222M0303, for the development and commercialization of police officers' life-log acquisition and stress/health management system through artificial intelligence based on big data analysis) funded by the Korean National Police Agency (KNPA, Seoul, Republic of Korea).

Institutional Review Board Statement: Not applicable.

Informed Consent Statement: Not applicable.

Data Availability Statement: Not applicable.

Conflicts of Interest: The authors declare no conflict of interest.

References

1. Slater, M.; Sanchez-Vives, M.V. Enhancing our lives with immersive virtual reality. *Front. Robot. AI* **2016**, *3*, 1–47. [CrossRef]
2. Slater, M. Immersion and the illusion of presence in virtual reality. *Brit. J. Psychol.* **2018**, *109*, 431–433. [CrossRef] [PubMed]
3. Emmelkamp, P.M.G.; Meyerbroker, K. Virtual reality therapy in mental health. *Annu. Rev. Clin. Psychol.* **2021**, *17*, 495–519. [CrossRef] [PubMed]
4. Cieslik, B.; Mazurek, J.; Rutkowski, S.; Kiper, P.; Turolla, A.; Szczepanska-Gieracha, J. Virtual reality in psychiatric disorders: A systematic review of reviews. *Complement. Ther. Med.* **2020**, *52*, 102480. [CrossRef] [PubMed]
5. Maples-Keller, J.L.; Yasinski, C.; Manjin, N.; Rothbaum, B.O. Virtual reality-enhanced extinction of phobias and post-traumatic stress. *Neurotherapeutics* **2017**, *14*, 554–563. [CrossRef] [PubMed]
6. Schiza, E.; Matsangidou, M.; Neokleous, K.; Pattichis, C.S. Virtual reality applications for neurological disease: A review. *Front. Robot. AI* **2019**, *6*, 100. [CrossRef]
7. Georgiev, D.D.; Georgieva, I.; Gong, Z.; Nanjappan, V.; Georgiev, G.V. Virtual reality for neurorehabilitation and cognitive enhancement. *Brain Sci.* **2021**, *11*, 221. [CrossRef]
8. Somrak, A.; Pogacnik, M.; Guna, J. Suitability and comparison of questionnaires assessing virtual reality-induced symptoms and effects and user experience in virtual environments. *Sensors* **2021**, *21*, 1185. [CrossRef]

9. Kim, H.K.; Park, J.; Choi, Y.; Choe, M. Virtual reality sickness questionnaire (VRSQ): Motion sickness measurement index in a virtual reality environment. *Appl. Ergon.* **2018**, *69*, 66–73. [CrossRef]
10. Aarsland, D.; Batzu, L.; Halliday, G.M.; Geurtsen, G.J.; Ballard, C.; Ray Chaudhuri, K.; Weintraub, D. Parkinson disease-associated cognitive impairment. *Nat. Rev. Dis. Primers* **2021**, *7*, 47. [CrossRef]
11. Arvanitakis, Z.; Shah, R.C.; Bennett, D.A. Diagnosis and management of dementia: Review. *JAMA* **2019**, *322*, 1589–1599. [CrossRef] [PubMed]
12. Pinto, T.C.C.; Machado, L.; Bulgacov, T.M.; Rodrigues-Junior, A.L.; Costa, M.L.G.; Ximenes, R.C.C.; Sougey, E.B. Is the Montreal Cognitive Assessment (MoCA) screening superior to the Mini-Mental State Examination (MMSE) in the detection of mild cognitive impairment (MCI) and Alzheimer's Disease (AD) in the elderly? *Int. Psychogeriatr.* **2019**, *31*, 491–504. [CrossRef] [PubMed]
13. Li, X.; Dai, J.; Zhao, S.; Liu, W.; Li, H. Comparison of the value of Mini-Cog and MMSE screening in the rapid identification of Chinese outpatients with mild cognitive impairment. *Medicine* **2018**, *97*, e10966. [CrossRef] [PubMed]
14. Shim, Y.S.; Yang, D.W.; Kim, H.J.; Park, Y.H.; Kim, S. Characteristic differences in the mini-mental state examination used in Asian countries. *BMC Neurol.* **2017**, *17*, 141. [CrossRef] [PubMed]
15. Liddell, T.M.; Kruschke, J.K. Analyzing ordinal data with metric models: What could possibly go wrong? *J. Exp. Soc. Psychol.* **2018**, *79*, 328–348. [CrossRef]
16. Kunz, L.; Schroder, T.N.; Lee, H.; Montag, C.; Lachmann, B.; Sariyska, R.; Reuter, M.; Stirnberg, R.; Stocker, T.; Messing-Floeter, P.C.; et al. Reduced grid-cell-like representations in adults at genetic risk for Alzheimer's disease. *Science* **2015**, *350*, 430–433. [CrossRef]
17. Moon, H.-J.; Gauthier, B.; Park, H.-D.; Faivre, N.; Blanke, O. Sense of self impacts spatial navigation and hexadirectional coding in human entorhinal cortex. *Commun. Biol.* **2022**, *5*, 406. [CrossRef]
18. Horing, B.; Newsome, N.D.; Enck, P.; Babu, S.V.; Muth, E.R. A virtual experimenter to increase standardization for the investigation of placebo effects. *BMC Med. Res. Methodol.* **2016**, *16*, 84. [CrossRef]
19. Ekstrom, A.D. Why vision is important to how we navigate. *Hippocampus* **2015**, *25*, 731–735. [CrossRef]
20. Engel, S.A.; Rumelhart, D.E.; Wandell, B.A.; Lee, A.T.; Glover, G.H.; Chichilnisky, E.J.; Shadlen, M.N. fMRI of human visual cortex. *Nature* **1994**, *369*, 525. [CrossRef]
21. Ba, F.; Sang, T.T.; He, W.; Fatehi, J.; Mostofi, E.; Zheng, B. Stereopsis and Eye Movement Abnormalities in Parkinson's Disease and Their Clinical Implications. *Front. Aging Neurosci.* **2022**, *14*, 783773. [CrossRef] [PubMed]
22. Alberts, J.L.; McGrath, M.; Miller Koop, M.; Waltz, C.; Scelina, L.; Scelina, K.; Rosenfeldt, A.B. The immersive cleveland clinic virtual reality shopping platform for the assessment of instrumental activities of daily living. *J. Vis. Exp.* **2022**, *preprint*. [CrossRef]
23. Petrigna, L.; Gentile, A.; Mani, D.; Pajaujiene, S.; Zanotto, T.; Thomas, E.; Paoli, A.; Palma, A.; Bianco, A. Dual-task conditions on static postural control in older adults: A systematic review and meta-analysis. *J. Aging Phys. Act.* **2021**, *29*, 162–177. [CrossRef] [PubMed]
24. Beauchet, O.; Dubost, V.; Allai, G.; Gonthier, R.; Hermann, F.R.; Kressig, R.W. 'Faster counting while walking' as a predictor of falls in older adults. *Age Ageing* **2007**, *36*, 418–423. [CrossRef] [PubMed]
25. Ehrsson, H.H. The experimental induction of out-of-body experiences. *Science* **2007**, *317*, 1048. [CrossRef] [PubMed]
26. Lenggenhager, B.; Tadi, T.; Metzinger, T.; Blanke, O. Video ergo sum: Manipulating bodily self-consciousness. *Science* **2007**, *317*, 1096–1099. [CrossRef] [PubMed]
27. De Ridder, D.; Van Laere, K.; Dupont, P.; Menovsky, T.; Van de Heyning, P. Visualizing out-of-body experience in the brain. *N. Engl. J. Med.* **2007**, *357*, 1829–1833. [CrossRef]
28. Ffytche, D.H.; Creese, B.; Politis, M.; Chaudhuri, K.R.; Weintraub, D.; Ballard, C.; Aarsland, D. The psychosis spectrum in Parkinson disease. *Nat. Rev. Neurol.* **2017**, *13*, 81–95. [CrossRef]
29. Bernasconi, F.; Blondiaux, E.; Potheegadoo, J.; Stripeikyte, G.; Pagonabarraga, J.; Bejr-Kasem, H.; Bassolino, M.; Akselrod, M.; Martinez-Horta, S.; Sampedro, F.; et al. Robot-induced hallucinations in Parkinson's disease depend on altered sensorimotor processing in fronto-temporal network. *Sci. Transl. Med.* **2021**, *13*, eabc8362. [CrossRef]
30. Stephenson, N. *Snow Crash*; Bantam Books: New York, NY, USA, 1992.
31. Petrigna, L.; Musumeci, G. The metaverse: A new challenge for the healthcare system: A scoping review. *J. Funct. Morphol. Kinesiol.* **2022**, *7*, 63. [CrossRef]
32. Hagerty, S.L.; Williams, L.M. The impact of COVID-19 on mental health: The interactive roles of brain biotypes and human connection. *Brain Behav. Immun. Health* **2020**, *5*, 100078. [CrossRef]
33. Li, Y.Y.; Godai, K.; Kido, M.; Komori, S.; Shima, R.; Kamide, K.; Kabayama, M. Cognitive decline and poor social relationship in older adults during COVID-19 pandemic: Can Information and Communications Technology (ICT) use helps? *BMC Geriatr.* **2022**, *22*, 375. [CrossRef] [PubMed]
34. Mace, R.A.; Mattos, M.K.; Vranceanu, A.M. Older adults can use technology: Why healthcare professionals must overcome ageism in digital health. *Transl. Behav. Med.* **2022**, *online ahead of print*. [CrossRef]
35. Marimuthu, R.; Gupta, S.; Stapleton, L.; Duncan, D.; Pasik-Duncan, B. Challenging the digital divide: Factors affecting the availability, adoption and acceptance of future technology in elderly user communities. *Computer* **2022**, *55*, 56–66. [CrossRef]

MDPI
St. Alban-Anlage 66
4052 Basel
Switzerland
Tel. +41 61 683 77 34
Fax +41 61 302 89 18
www.mdpi.com

Brain Sciences Editorial Office
E-mail: brainsci@mdpi.com
www.mdpi.com/journal/brainsci

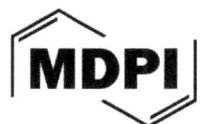

www.ingramcontent.com/pod-product-compliance
Lightning Source LLC
LaVergne TN
LVHW070606100526
838202LV00012B/577